THE FLORIDA SENIOR LEGAL GUIDE
NINTH EDITION

LEGAL
HEALTH
ESTATE PLANNING

GREGORY G. GAY
MEMBER OF THE FLORIDA BAR

SENIOR LAW SERIES, INC.

Publisher's Cataloging-in-Publication
(Provided by Quality Books, Inc.)

Gay, Gregory G.
    The Florida senior legal guide : legal, health,
estate planning / Gregory G. Gay. -- Ninth edition.
    pages cm
    Includes index.
    ISBN 978-1-929397-04-4
    ISBN 978-1-929397-05-1 (ebook)

    1. Older people--Legal status, laws, etc.--Florida--
Popular works. 2. Estate planning--Florida--Popular
works. 3. Health planning--Law and legislation--Florida
--Popular works.   I. Title.

    KFF91.A3G39 2015   346.75901'3
                    QBI15-600036

ISBN 978-1-929397-07-5 (First Edition)
ISBN 978-1-929397-08-2 (Second Edition)
ISBN 978-1-929397-10-5 (Third Edition)
ISBN 978-1-929397-09-9 (Fourth Edition)
ISBN 978-1-929397-13-6 (Fifth Edition)
ISBN 978-1-929397-14-3 (Sixth Edition)
ISBN 978-1-929397-15-0 (Sixth Edition - ebook)
ISBN 978-1-929397-00-6 (Seventh Edition)
ISBN 978-1-929397-01-3 (Seventh Edition - ebook)
ISBN 978-1-929397-02-0 (Eighth Edition)
ISBN 978-1-929397-03-7 (Eighth Edition - ebook)
ISBN 978-1-929397-04-4 (Ninth Edition)
ISBN 978-1-929397-05-1 (Ninth Edition - ebook)

Inquiries should be addressed to:
Senior Law Series, Inc. P.O. Box 733
New Port Richey, Florida 34656-0733

Interior design and typesetting by Digital Publishing of Florida, Inc.
Cover design by George Foster

DEDICATION

To Julia,

The love of my life.

ABOUT THE AUTHOR

Gregory G. Gay, Esq. is the President of the Nature Coast Law Offices of Gregory G. Gay, P.A. that has law offices in New Port Richey, Spring Hill and Crystal River, Florida. Mr. Gay was admitted to the Florida Bar in 1973. Mr. Gay is Board Certified by the Florida Bar's Board of Legal Specialization in Wills, Trusts & Estates and in Elder Law. He is also Board Certified in Elder Law by the National Elder Law Foundation and is designated by that organization as a Certified Advanced Practitioner. Mr. Gay is also a Florida Supreme Court certified civil court mediator. Mr. Gay received his Bachelor of Science Degree in Accounting and a Juris Doctor Degree from Florida State University. He has also earned a Master of Science Degree in Financial Services from The American College, a Master of Arts Degree in Biblical Studies from Dallas Theological Seminary and a Master of Divinity Degree from Southeastern Baptist Theological Seminary. Mr. Gay is a Director of The Florida Lawyers' Legal Insurance Corporation. Mr. Gay is a past President of the Tampa Bay Planned Giving Council and is a past President of the North Suncoast Estate Planning Council. Mr. Gay is a past president of the West Pasco Bar Association. He is also a past Chairman of the Pasco Hernando State College Board of Trustees. Mr. Gay is a past President of the New Port Richey Rotary Club and has been awarded a Paul Harris Fellow by this club. Mr. Gay is a member of Idelwild Baptist Church in Tampa, Florida. Mr. Gay serves on the Board of Directors of Living Water Community Tranformation, Inc. that enriches the lives of the people of the community of Akot, South Sudan, both spiritually and through the education of their children. Mr. Gay is also a Director of the Community Aging and Retirement Services, Inc. (CARES) that provides needed services to seniors in Pasco County, Florida. He is married to Julia Stokes from Miami and they have two adult children and one grandson.

Table of Contents

Page

Preface x

PART ONE
Planning for Retirement

Chapter 1 **SOCIAL SECURITY** 3
An Overview of the National Social Security Program 3
Social Security Taxes and Limits on Earnings 4
Regular Retirement 6
Early Retirement 6
Late Retirement 8
Taxation of Social Security Benefits 9
Benefits for a Married Spouse of a Retired Worker 10
Benefits for a Divorced Spouse of a Retired Worker 10
Surviving Spouse's Benefits 11
Family Benefits for a Deceased Worker 11
Parent's Benefits 12
Disability Benefits and Eligibility 12
Determining Disability 13
Working While Receiving Disability Benefits 13
Disabled Widow's/Widower's Benefits 13
Family Benefits for a Disabled Worker 14

Chapter 2 **MEDICARE** 15
Medicare Part A 16
Hospital Care 16
Skilled Nursing Facility Care 18
Home Health Care 18
Hospice 20
Medicare Part B 21
Qualified Medicare Beneficiary 23
Specified Low Income Medicare Beneficiary 23
Medigap Insurance Policy 24
Medicare Advantage 25
Medicare Part D 26

Chapter 3 **TAXATION OF PENSION PLAN**
AND IRA DISTRIBUTIONS 29
Distribution of Pension Plan Benefits 29

Premature Distributions 30
Required Distributions... 31
Distributions During the Participant's Lifetime..................... 32
Distributions Upon Participant's Death
      Before Required Beginning Date 32
Distributions Upon Participant's Death
      After Required Beginning Date 32
Rollover by Surviving Spouse.. 33
Inherited IRA.. 33
Trust As Beneficiary 36
Roth IRA.. 37
IRA Contribution Limit.. 38
Estate Taxation of IRA 40

Chapter 4   **ANNUITIES** 41
Definitions... 41
Death of Owner.. 42
Death of the Annuitant... 42
Types of Annuities.. 43
Immediate Annuities.. 43
Life Income Annuity.. 43
Life with Period Certain... 43
Deferred Annuities 44
Free Look Period 45
Penalty for Early Withdrawal.. 45
Income Taxation of Annuities 45
Distribution at Death... 47
Inappropriate Sale Practices 47
Estate Taxation of Annuities... 49

Chapter 5   **SELLING A RESIDENCE AND HOMESTEAD EXEMPTIONS** 51
Capital Gain Exclusion on the Sale of a Residence 51
Reverse Mortgage 52
Florida Documentary Stamp Tax 54
Title Insurance 55
Property Tax Exemptions.. 56

PART TWO
Planning for Disability

Chapter 6   **OVERVIEW OF HEALTH CARE ADVANCE DIRECTIVES** 59

Chapter 7   **LIVING WILLS** 61
Living Will 61
Terminal Condition, Persistent Vegetative State
      and End-Stage Condition 61
Definition of Life-Prolonging Procedure................................. 62
Elective Procedures... 62
Procedure for Exercising a Living Will...................................... 62

Procedure in Absence of a Living Will 63
Effect of Living Wills Made Prior to October 1, 1999 64
Prohibition of Mercy Killing 65

Chapter 8   **HEALTH CARE SURROGATE DESIGNATION** 69

Chapter 9   **DO-NOT-RESUSCITATE ORDER** 71

Chapter 10   **ABSENCE OF ADVANCE DIRECTIVES** 73

Chapter 11   **DURABLE POWER OF ATTORNEY** 75

Chapter 12   **PLANNING FOR PETS** 79

Chapter 13   **BAKER ACT** 81
Baker Act 81
Guardian Advocate for Baker Act Proceedings 83

Chapter 14   **GUARDIANSHIPS** 85

Chapter 15   **DEVELOPMENTAL DISABILITIES** 89

Chapter 16   **ADULT FAMILY-CARE HOMES** 93

Chapter 17   **NURSING HOME PATIENT RIGHTS** 95
Nursing Home Discharges 95
Resident's Rights 97
Office of the Local Long-Term Care Ombudsman 98
Selecting a Nursing Home 98

Chapter 18   **ELDER ABUSE** 99

Chapter 19   **MEDICAID NURSING HOME ASSISTANCE** 103
Eligibility 103
Non-Countable Assets 104
Lady Bird Deed 106
Transferring Assets 107
Promissory Notes, Loans and Mortgages 108
Undue Hardship 108
Irrevocable Annuities 108
Half-A-Loaf 110
Personal Service Contract 110
Exemptions to the Transfer Rules 112
Supplemental Needs Trusts and Pooled Trusts 112
Assisted Living Facility Medicaid Waiver Program 114
Medicaid Estate Recovery 116
Medicaid Managed Care 117
Just Say No 118

Chapter 20 LONG-TERM CARE INSURANCE 121

    Long-Term Care Insurance 121

    Long-Term Care Insurance Partnership Program 123

Chapter 21 LIFE CARE PLANNING 125

Chapter 22 ELDER MEDIATION and SHARED FAMILY DECISION MAKING 127

Chapter 23 VIATICAL AND LIFE SETTLEMENT AGREEMENTS 129

Chapter 24 GRANDPARENT VISITATION 131

Part Three
Estate Planning

Chapter 25 WILLS 135

Chapter 26 TRUSTS 139

    Revocable Trust 139

    Irrevocable Trust 141

    Florida's Trust Code 142

Chapter 27 PRENUPTIAL AGREEMENTS 145

Chapter 28 FLORIDA'S ELECTIVE ESTATE 147

Chapter 29 FEDERAL ESTATE AND GIFT TAX LAW 149

    Federal Estate and Gift Tax Laws 149

    Federal Estate Tax Return 150

    No Florida Estate Tax 150

    Determining the Gross Estate 150

    Basis in Property Received From a Decedent Who Dies in 2015 151

    Basis In Property Received During His or Her Lifetime 151

    Portability of Unused Exemption Between Spouses 152

    Gift Tax Annual Exclusion 154

Chapter 30 CHARITABLE GIVING 155

    Deductions for Present Contributions 155

    Deferred Giving 156

    Charitable Remainder Trust 157

    Charitable Lead Trust 159

    Gift Annuities 159

    Pooled Income Fund 160

Chapter 31 PROBATE 161

    Personal Representatives Compensation 162

    Attorney Fees 162

    Alternatives to Formal Probate 163

     Summary Administration...164
     Disposition without Need of Administration..164
     Automobile 164
     Homestead 165

Chapter 32 **ARRANGING THE FUNERAL**..167
     Pre-Need Arrangements 167
     Cremation..168
     The Need for Written Funeral Instructions 169
     Organ Donation 170

Chapter 33 **VETERANS BENEFITS** 173
     Overview of Veterans Benefits..173
     Compensation 173
     Non-Service Connected Pension...174
     Medical Care..176
     Geriatric Services 176
     Prescription Benefits...177

Chapter 34 **VETERANS CEMETERIES** 179
     Veterans Cemeteries 179

Chapter 35 **PATIENT PROTECTION AND AFFORDABLE CARE ACT** 181
     Overview of the Patient and Affordable Care Act 181
     Young Adult Coverage...181
     Unlimited Coverage 182
     Pre-Existing Condition..182
     Non-Rescission..182
     Non-Discrimination...182
     Required Coverage 182
     The Penalty 182
     The Health Insurance Exchange 183
     Premium Tax Credit 184
     Legal Challenges to Affordable Care Act 184
     First Challenge...184
     Second Challenge...185

Chapter 36 **RECOGNITION OF SAME-SEX MARRIAGE FOR
              PURPOSES OF FEDERAL LAW AND FLORIDA LAW**................187
     Recognition of Same-Sex Marriage for Purposes of Federal Law
         and Regulations 187
     Recognition of Same-Sex Marriage for Purposes of Florida Law....................190
     Supreme Court of United States to Review Circuit Split.................................191

     Glossary 193

     Index 205

PREFACE

The number of "senior citizens" is rapidly increasing. Presently, at least 7,000 Baby Boomers attain age 65 every day. During the next 18 years, there may be as many as 10,000 Baby Boomers attaining age 65 each day. Four million and six hundred thousand of these boomers now reside in Florida. Florida is the fourth largest boomer state in the nation.

The senior citizen population is projected to grow from 40.7 million in the year 2010 to 76.3 million in 2030. The U.S. Census Bureau projects that our American population age 85 and over could grow from 5.3 million in 2006 to nearly 21 million in the year 2050. However, 13.5 million people are predicted to have Alzheimer's disease by 2050 unless a cure is found.

Three out of four seniors now begin claiming Social Security early retirement benefits the moment they are eligible at age 62. Most are doing this out of necessity. However, by claiming Social Security early, they will be locked in at a much lower amount of Social Security income than if they waited until regular retirement at age 66 or late retirement at age 70.

The 2014 Annual Report of the Board of Trustees of the Federal Old-Age and Survivors Insurance and Federal Disability Insurance Trust Funds reports that "Neither Medicare nor Social Security can sustain projected long-run program costs in full under currently scheduled financing, and legislative changes are necessary to avoid disruptive consequences for beneficiaries and taxpayers." Social Security and Medicare together accounted for 41 percent of Federal expenditures in fiscal year 2013. In addition, the Trustees project the disability income trust fund's depletion late in 2016. Lawmakers need to act soon to avoid automatic reductions in payments to Disability Income beneficiaries in late 2016.

The Trustees project that the Medicare Hospital Insurance (HI) Trust Fund will be the next to face depletion after the Disability Income Trust Fund. The projected date of Medicare Hospital Insurance Trust Fund's depletion is 2030. At that time dedicated revenues will be sufficient to only pay 85 percent of Medicare Hospital Insurance costs.

Fortunately, the Trustees project that Part B of Supplementary Medical Insurance (SMI), which pays doctors' bills and other outpatient expenses, and Part D, which provides access to prescription drug coverage, will remain adequately financed into the indefinite future because current law automatically provides financing each year to meet the next year's expected costs.

This Commission concludes by stating that lawmakers should address the financial challenges facing Social Security and Medicare as soon as possible. Taking action sooner rather than later will leave more options and more time available to phase in changes so that the public has adequate time to prepare.

The amount of assets that a person can leave at death without a federal estate tax has increased to $5.43 million. The annual gift tax exclusion will remain at $14,000 per donee in 2015. The Internal Revenue Service's new regulations permit minimum distributions from an Individual Retirement Account until age 115.

Another change relates to the fact that there are now five groups of "senior citizens." A person in the youngest age group referred to as "senior citizens" was born between 1950 and 1960. This boomer often looks at the other customer in the check-out line when asked if he or she intends to accept the senior citizen discount. This most recent age group of senior citizens will need to reconsider the concept of retirement. The Social Security regular retirement age is increasing. A person retiring at age 62 in the year 2015 will only receive 75 percent of the regular retirement benefit that would be paid at age 66.

The senior citizen born between 1940 and 1949 rarely thinks of himself or herself as old. Now, only the extended weekends (Friday to Sunday) are filled with golfing, fishing, bridge and exercise. The continuing of the vocation from Monday to Thursday provides the needed supplemental income. Numerous week-long vacations for cruising and sight-seeing are foremost. These seniors are truly spending their children's inheritance. The senior citizen born during these years is experiencing a need for a second round of estate planning. Due to the increase in the federal estate tax exclusion to $5.43 million, a person this age must reconsider the previous need for a his and her credit shelter bypass trust since this may unnecessarily deprive the surviving spouse of a total inheritance. In addition, the purchase of long-term care insurance or establishing a side-fund for this reality is now essential.

A senior citizen born between 1930 and 1939 is truly unique. He or she is part of the fastest growing generation. At this age, every year of life results in the loss of only 3/10th of a year on Social Security's life-expectancy tables. But, the cost to maintain and insure the homestead as well as the summer home is no longer economically viable.

For a senior citizen born before 1930, quality of life is not merely a phrase; it is the thing hoped for. A person living beyond age 85 experiences a one-in-two chance of developing Alzheimer's disease or another form of dementia. Life-prolonging procedures and expensive long-term care alternatives are desired by persons of this age group only if there will then be a meaningful existence. Equally important, a person of this generation feels a responsibility to leave something to his or her children in case there is another economic disaster on the scale of the Great Depression through which he or she suffered.

Those who do retire must remember that they are Biblically admonished to visit the sick, true widows and orphans. If physically able, evangelizing and mission work is Biblically instructed. So, do not just plan to retire. Plan to retire to some enjoyable and meaningful vocation.

But, the story does not end with seniors attaining age 86. A few years ago, a client asked me how to invest the proceeds she received from the life insurance company that paid all the policy benefits to her because she attained age 100. She died this year, having attained the age of 109. There will be many people living beyond age 100. How our nation treats this new and unexpected generation of senior citizens will define its character.

Nearly one-half of the Boomers attaining age 66 this year may not have enough savings to cover basic living expenses. Most of these persons only have $60,000 in savings. Fortunately, two-thirds of these retiring boomers will receive an inheritance from their parents. However, the median amount of this inheritance will be $64,000. It is estimated that only 13% of those turning 66 this year plan to retire completely in 2015. Nearly 24% don't know when they will retire. Another 40% of this age group plan to work until they die. It is important to understand that continuing to work beyond age 66 is not all bad. A trade-off of a continued busy work life will be more meaningful than hours of boredom. Just think of what Bobby Bowden accomplished and the number of athletes he inspired and trained to become professional athletes after he attained age 66.

The Florida Senior Legal Guide 9th Edition will assist persons from each of these age groups by explaining the laws especially affecting senior citizens. An informed senior citizen can then make better and more informed decisions regarding complex legal issues that arise in these later stages of life.

Finally, this book is also intended as a reference guide for our youth and caregivers to help them better understand the legal complexities and challenges facing today's senior citizens.

PART ONE
PLANNING FOR RETIREMENT

CHAPTER 1

SOCIAL SECURITY

- An Overview of the National Social Security Program
- Social Security Taxes and Limits on Earnings
- Regular Retirement
- Early Retirement
- Late Retirement
- Taxation of Social Security Benefits
- Benefits for a Married Spouse of a Retired Worker
- Benefits for a Divorced Spouse of a Retired Worker
- Surviving Spouse's Benefits
- Family Benefits for a Deceased Worker
- Parent's Benefits
- Disability Benefits and Eligibility
- Determining Disability
- Working While Receiving Disability Benefits
- Disabled Widow's/Widower's Benefits
- Family Benefits for a Disabled Worker

An Overview of the National Social Security Program

Presently, about 64 million people collect some form of Social Security benefit. Fifty-eight million people receive retirement benefits. An additional eight million people receive Social Security Disability Income known as SSDI. Social Security originated as a retirement program. However, today's Social Security system provides much more. Persons other than retirees receiving benefits are the disabled, spouses and dependents of persons who receive Social Security, widows, widowers and children of deceased workers. Thus, depending on the circumstances, a person may be eligible for Social Security at any age.

The contributions from the Social Security tax presently paid by in excess of 168 million employees are sufficient at this time to pay the benefits received by the retired and disabled workers and still create a reserve. However, several years ago, Congress recognized that the pay-as-you-go Social Security system will be insufficient in future years to fund the increased demand for benefits brought about by the increasing number of retired workers.

In 1950, the ratio of workers to beneficiaries was 16 to 1. Presently, there are 3 workers for every Social Security beneficiary. By the time the Boomer generation attains full retirement age, this ratio will be 2.1 workers for every 1 beneficiary. By 2030, the Baby Boomer generation will double the number of retirees receiving Social Security benefits. In recognition of these demographic changes, Congress passed legislation a few years ago intended to respond to this increasing demand for retirement benefits.

The legislation increases "Full retirement age" for workers born in 1943 or later. Full retirement age now caps at age 67 for workers born after 1959. Thus, baby boomers will have to wait longer to receive their regular old-age Social Security benefits.

Year of Birth		Full Retirement Age
1943-1954		66
1955		66 and 2 months
1956		66 and 4 months
1957		66 and 6 months
1958		66 and 8 months
1959		66 and 10 months
1960 and later		67

Social Security Taxes and Limits on Earnings

The percentage of Social Security tax that will be deducted from a worker's pay in 2015 is 6.2 percent of earnings. It is estimated that the social security tax will be paid by 168 million workers in 2015. The maximum amount on which this tax is imposed for the year 2015 will be $118,500. The maximum that can be withheld from a worker for the social security tax in 2015 will be $7,347.00. The percentage of Social Security tax and the maximum amount of earnings on which this tax is imposed may increase each year. Employers will also pay an additional 6.2% of their employees' covered wages in 2015 for their share of social security taxes. Self-employed individuals will pay 12.4% of their income in social security taxes up to the $118,500 wage base. A Medicare tax is also deducted from a worker's paycheck. Presently, this is 1.45% of earnings for employees earning less than $200,000. There is an additional Medicare Tax for single workers earning more than $200,000. Married couples filing a joint return who earn more than $250,000 will have to pay this additional Medicare Tax. The rate of the additional Medicare Tax is 0.9% on the wages in excess of $200,000. This statute requires an employer to withhold the additional Medicare Tax on wages or compensation the employer pays to an employee in excess of $200,000 in a calendar year. An employer has this withholding obligation even though an employee may not be liable for the

Additional Medicare Tax because, for example, the employee's wages or other compensation together with that of his or her spouse (when filing a joint return) does not exceed the $250,000 liability threshold. Any withheld but unassessed Additional Medicare Tax will be credited against the total tax liability shown on the individual's income tax return (Form 1040). The employer is not required to notify an employee when it begins withholding the Additional Medicare Tax. There is no employer match for the Additional Medicare Tax. An example for a single taxpayer with wages of $245,000 is as follows. In 2015, a single individual with wages of $245,000 will owe the Medicare tax rate of 1.45% on the first $200,000 of wages. The Medicare higher rate of 2.35% will be applied to the remaining $45,000 of wages for 2015. Employers will be responsible for collecting and remitting the additional Medicare payroll tax on wages that exceed $200,000. There is no maximum amount of earnings on which this tax is imposed.

A surtax in addition to the federal income tax is imposed on the net investment income of individuals, estates and trusts. This is commonly referred to as the Medicare tax. This surtax for individuals is 3.8% of the lesser of the taxpayer's modified adjusted gross income in excess of the threshold amount or the taxpayer's net investment income for that year. The threshold amount is $200,000 for individuals, $250,000 for married couples or $125,000 for married taxpayers filing separately. This threshold amount is not indexed for inflation.

Net investment income includes gross income from interest, dividends, rents, royalties, annuities, gains from the disposition of property, passive activities less allocable expenses. Capital gains are an item of net investment income. However, several types of income are specifically excluded from the definition of investment income. They include distributions from IRAs and qualified plans, non-passive trade or business income, tax-exempt income, tax-exempt annuities and income subject to self-employment tax. Rental income is generally passive and counted toward net investment income. However, there is an exception for real estate professionals that devote 750 hours or more each year to working in the real estate business.

There is also a net investment income tax on estates and trusts equal to 3.8% of the lesser of the estate's or trust's adjusted gross income in excess of the highest income tax bracket threshold which is $12,300 for 2015, or the estate's or trust's undistributed net investment income. Distributions from an estate or trust reduce the income subject to the 3.8% tax on net investment income. The threshold for estates and trusts is indexed for inflation.

Until the Net Investment Income and other income reach the threshold applicable to the taxpayer, the surtax is not triggered. Once the other income and the net investment income exceed the threshold amount, only the excess over the threshold amount is subject to the surtax.

The Senior Citizens Freedom to Work Act eliminated the Social Security retirement earnings test in and after the month in which a person reaches regular retirement age. However, the Senior Citizens Freedom to Work Act does not repeal the present maximum that can be earned without a reduction in Social Security benefits between ages 62 and 66. The maximum amount that a worker under age 66 can earn without a reduction in Social Security benefits in the year 2015 will be $15,772. The maximum that can be earned without a reduction in Social Security benefits may be adjusted by Congress each year. For every $2 earned over the limit, $1 is withheld from Social Security benefits. However, during the calendar year in which a worker born in 1949 attains age 66, the amount that can be earned prior to his or her birth month without reduction in Social Security benefits in the year 2015 is 3,490 per month. For every $3 earned over this limit, there is a $1 withheld. A person can earn an unlimited amount of income without a penalty after attaining age 66. Only wages and net self-employment income count toward the Social Security earnings limit. Income from savings, investments, interest, pensions, annuities, capital gains or insurance will not affect a retired worker's benefits. Failure to inform the Social Security Administration of any excess earnings by April 15th of the year following the excess earnings may result in the imposition of an additional penalty.

Regular Retirement

A wage earner today may take normal retirement and begin receiving monthly Social Security checks at age 66 if born between 1943 and 1954 (see chart on Page 4). At least 40 quarters of credit for contributing to Social Security (ten years of work) are needed to qualify for Social Security benefits. The amount of earnings upon which Social Security is paid in order to earn a quarter of coverage from wages or net income in the year 2015 is $1,220. A credit is earned by reporting at least $1,220 in 2015 of wages or net income from self- employment at any time in a year. Thus, a worker can receive credit for four quarters in a year by earning the $4,880 ($1,202 x 4= $4,880) at any time during a year. This minimum amount of earnings for credit for a quarter of coverage increases each year.

Early Retirement

A person may still elect to start receiving Social Security benefits as early as age 62 at a reduced rate. Since the minimum retirement age remains at 62 but the regular retirement age has increased, a person retiring early must understand that there will be a reduced monthly benefit. For example, a person who has a full retirement age of 67 and retires at age 62 will have his or her benefit reduced 5/9 of 1 percent for each of the 36 months between age 64 and age 67 plus 5/12 of 1 percent for each month in excess of 36 months before normal retirement age. Thus, if this person whose normal retirement would have been age 67 retires early at age

62, he or she will only receive 70 percent of his or her full retirement benefit.

The disadvantage to taking early retirement is that it will permanently reduce a worker's monthly benefit. Thus, if a worker eligible for regular retirement at age 66 chooses early retirement at age 62 and lives beyond age 77, the worker may ultimately receive less in total benefits.

In addition, a surviving spouse may receive less social security benefits for the rest of his or her lifetime due to early retirement. This is because the survivor can receive his or her own benefit or the deceased spouse's benefit, whichever is more. If the deceased spouse had a larger benefit than the surviving spouse, the surviving spouse will be limited to his or her smaller benefit or the reduced benefit paid to the deceased spouse who took early retirement.

LIFE SITUATION #1

John, who was 62 in January of 2015, is considering early retirement. John would receive $1,000 per month at normal retirement. John wants to know how much he would lose in Social Security benefits over his lifetime if he retires at age 62, rather than the normal retirement age of 66. John is in good health and both of his parents lived until age 85. John will only receive 75 percent of his normal retirement benefit if he retires at age 62. This is because his benefit will be reduced 5/9 of 1 percent for each of the 36 months between age 63 and age 66 plus 5/12 of 1 percent for each month in excess of 36 months before normal retirement age. The following chart shows the total Social Security benefits John will receive at various points following retirement, depending on whether John retires at the normal retirement age of 66 or takes early retirement at age 62.

Year	Last month of age	Retirement at 62 Total Benefit is 75% of Annual Benefit Selected	Retirement at age 66 Total Benefit is 100% of Annual Benefit Selected
2015	62	$ 9,000	----------
2019	66	$45,000	$ 12,000
2023	70	$81,000	$ 60,000
2026	74	$117,000	$108,000
2030	78	$153,000	$158,000
2034	82	$189,000	$206,000
2038	86	$225,000	$254,000
2042	90	$263,000	$302,000

The breakeven point is during the 16th year after early retirement at age 62. At this point, the total benefit for the person who selected normal retirement exceeds the total benefit for the person who selected early retirement. Since it is assumed for the purpose of this illustration that the monthly benefit will be used for living expenses, no projections have been made to determine how much the early retirement benefits might earn if they were invested for the entire period. In addition, the person who elects early retirement must not earn more than $15,772 per year between ages 62 and 65 without having to repay some of the social security received during the early retirement years.

Until 2011, persons turning age 62, could take an early Social Security retirement and then invest these funds until age 66. Then, the funds could be paid back to the Social Security Administration and a benefit at the normal retirement amount could be taken. This loophole has been eliminated as of 2011. Now, a person taking early retirement cannot pay back the previously withdrawn funds and begin receiving regular retirement benefits.

Late Retirement

A worker may find it advantageous to delay normal retirement in two ways. First, the extra income earned after full retirement age usually increases average earnings because the earnings in later years may be higher and will replace a previous lower year of earnings. The higher the earnings, the higher the monthly Social Security benefits. Secondly, a special credit is given to a worker who delays retirement. This credit is a percentage added on to the worker's Social Security benefit that varies depending on his or her full retirement age.

A delayed retirement credit of 8% per year is given for retirement after the normal retirement age. To receive this credit, a person must be working at his or her normal retirement age. No additional credit is given after age 70.

A person born in 1948 who intends to retire at age 70 would first determine his or her normal retirement age from the table on page 4. This person's normal retirement age is 66. The delayed retirement percentage for a person born in 1948 which is 8% per year would be multiplied by 4 for the additional years to be worked beyond normal retirement. Thus, the worker's benefit at age 70 would be 32% higher than his or her primary insurance amount at age 66.

A married worker who intends to take advantage of the late-retirement benefit may wish to consider filing for social security benefits at the full retirement age of 66, and then immediately suspend the receipt of his or her social security benefit until age 70 if the spouse's lifetime earnings are lower. If the spouse with the higher earnings record files for regular social security benefits at age 66 and then suspends his or her benefit, the spouse with the lower lifetime earnings may receive a higher normal retirement benefit based on the non-retiring spouse's record. This is because the spousal benefit is 50% of what his or her spouse is to receive at regular retirement. By example, John has reached full retirement age of 66, but intends to not receive Social Security benefits until age 70. His regular retirement monthly benefit is $1,800. By waiting until age 70 to begin receiving benefits, his monthly delayed retirement benefit will be 32% more or $2,376. If his wife, Mary, who is also age 66, has lower life-time earnings that will entitle her to only receive $750 per month from Social Security, she could instead request to receive at age 66 an amount equal to $900 per month, which is 50% of John's regular retirement benefit. However, John must first file for benefits at age 66 and then immediately suspend the receipt of the benefits. In addition, if John dies first after attaining age 70, Mary's benefit will increase to $2,376 per month. This is because her retirement benefit is based on the worker's benefit or his or her spouse's benefit, whichever is greater.

Taxation of Social Security Benefits

Presently, up to 85 percent of Social Security benefits may be included in taxable income if a taxpayer's income exceeds a certain amount. If an individual's gross income (including social security, taxable and tax exempt income) exceeds $25,000, he or she may be taxed on up to 85% of his or her Social Security benefits. A married couple, filing jointly, may be taxed on up to 85% of their Social Security benefit if their total gross income exceeds $32,000. There is no higher exclusion amount for a married person filing separately. Instead, the threshold will be $25,000. The calculation of the income tax on Social Security Benefits is explained in the following chart.

LIFE SITUATION #2

Gregory and Julia are age 66, and are married and retired. In the year 2015, they will receive $27,000 in investment earnings; $60,000 from Gregory and Julia's combined pension plan retirement benefits and $30,000 in combined Social Security retirement benefits. The amount of their Social Security that is subject to federal income tax is computed as follows:

1. Determine the taxpayer's modified adjusted gross income:
   Investment earnings $27,000
   plus: Pension benefits 60,000
   plus: one-half of Social Security benefits 15,000
   102,000

2. Determine the modified adjusted gross
   income over the first threshold: 102,000
   ($25,000 for singles; $32,000 for husband
   and wife filing jointly) (32,000)
   70,000

3. Determine the modified Adjusted Gross
   Income over the second threshold:
   Modified Adjusted Gross Income $102,000
   ($34,000 for singles; $44,000 for joint filers)   (44,000)   58,000

4. Determine the lesser of:
   a. One-half of the excess over the first threshold: $35,000
      Plus 35 percent of the excess over
      second threshold   20,300
                                                55,300
   b. 85 percent of Social Security benefit
                                                25,500
   c. 50 percent of total Social Security benefit   15,000
      plus 85 percent of excess over second threshold 49,300   64,300

Since the smallest of these three figures is $25,500, this is the amount of Social Security benefits that will be subject to income taxation.

Benefits for a Married Spouse of a Retired Worker

A spouse may receive up to a maximum of one-half of a retired or disabled worker's primary insurance amount subject to the family maximum. At age 62, the spouse's benefit would be 38.35 percent of the primary insurance amount. The spouse must have been married to the worker for at least one year and be at least 62 years of age. The spouse cannot be entitled to a higher old-age or disability benefit from his or her own record. Medicare benefits begin for a spouse at age 65.

Benefits for a Divorced Spouse of a Retired Worker

A divorced spouse is entitled to a monthly benefit equal to one-half of an insured's unreduced retirement amount. The divorced spouse must be at least 62 years of age, have been married to the worker for at least ten years and the couple must have been divorced for at least two years. This two-year wait is intended to discourage couples from divorcing in order for one member to receive benefits while the other continues to work. In addition, the divorced spouse cannot be remarried and cannot be entitled to a larger benefit on his or her account. An eligible divorced spouse will receive a further reduction if he or she retires before his or her full retirement age. The difference between the current spouse and a divorced spouse is that the current spouse cannot receive benefits on the worker's record until the worker actually files for Social Security benefits, whereas the divorced spouse may file for benefits once he or she meets the eligibility requirements and the worker is of retirement age (at least age 62). Medicare benefits begin for a divorced spouse at age 65.

Surviving Spouse's Benefits

A surviving spouse of a deceased worker who remains unmarried and has no dependent children under age 18 may retire and begin receiving a widow(er)'s benefits at 60, or 50 if disabled. The surviving spouse must have been married to the deceased wage earner for at least nine months. If the marriage was less than nine months, it must be proven that the deceased was reasonably expected to have lived nine months and that the insured's death was not expected. Medicare benefits begin for a widowed spouse at age 65. A subsequent marriage after age 60 will not affect the right to receive social security as the widow or widower of a deceased spouse. If a widow or widower remarries before age 60, there is no right to social security due to the death of the previous spouse. However, entitlement may again be considered if the current marriage ends in divorce or the current spouse dies.

The surviving spouse will also receive a lump sum death benefit of $255. This is a small stipend in relation to the actual cost of burial, which Florida's legislature has recognized as being on the average of $6,000.

Family Benefits for a Deceased Worker

If a spouse dies fully insured, the surviving spouse and the minor children are entitled to survivor's benefits. The surviving mother or father will receive Social Security benefits as a parent of a minor child until that child reaches the age of 16, or is over 16 and disabled and in the care of this parent. A child of the deceased worker will receive Social Security benefits until 18 as long as he or she remains unmarried. A child's benefits can continue to age 19 if he or she is attending a full-time secondary school. A child cannot be married and continue to receive benefits unless he or she is an adult disabled child who marries another dependent or survivor beneficiary.

These family benefits are subject to a family maximum. This means that although the surviving spouse and the minor children of a deceased worker may all be entitled to social security, there is a limit on how much a family may receive. The family maximum is never large enough to pay full benefits to more than two persons. The surviving mother or father and each child receive a proportionate share of this benefit. For example, if the family maximum due to the death of the father is $1,500 per month, then the mother and the three minor children would receive $375 each per month. It is also important to remember that the widow or widower and the minor children are not entitled to Medicare unless they are disabled. Thus, it maybe necessary to use a portion of this monthly Social Security family benefit for the family's health insurance premiums.

Parent's Benefits

A parent may be dependent on a worker at the time of the worker's death. This occurs if the parent is at least 62 years of age, receiving at least one-half of his or her support from the worker at the time of the worker's death, and is not entitled to his or her own Social Security benefit that exceeds the benefit to be received as a parent. The parent cannot be married when he or she applies for the benefit. However, the parent can subsequently marry another survivor or dependent after the benefit begins to be paid.

Disability Benefits and Eligibility

In order to receive Social Security Disability Insurance (SSDI), a worker must be under age 65 and have obtained a status of disability insured or specially insured. A worker meets the definition of disability-insured if he or she has enough credits of coverage during a certain period of time before becoming disabled. A credit is earned when a worker receives at least a minimum amount of earnings (presently $1,220 in 2015) during a quarter of a calendar year. However, a worker can earn 4 credits for a year by earning the minimum amount for the year at any time during the year. The worker must have credits for at least 20 quarters during the past 40-quarter period that ends with the quarter in which the disability occurred. This is referred to as the 20/40 rule. A person who is disabled due to blindness is not required to meet this 20/40 rule.

> **LIFE SITUATION #3:**
> A married mother with children 5 and 7 years old becomes disabled. She had worked the first five years of marriage and then stayed home the next seven years to raise the children. To receive any kind of benefit from the Social Security Administration, a wage earner must have worked at least five of the last ten years. In this case, the mother is not entitled to Social Security disability benefits. Had she worked part-time and earned enough to gain four quarters of coverage each year, she would be eligible. Example: for the year 2015, $1,220 in earnings equals one quarter of coverage. Therefore, $4,880 earned equals four quarters of coverage for 2015.

The exception to this disability-insured status rule relates to younger workers. For instance, a younger worker who has not worked long enough to meet the disability insured status may still be specially insured and entitled to disability benefits if he or she becomes disabled after age 21 and before age 31 and has credit for one-half the quarters from the time he or she attained age 21 until becoming disabled, with a minimum of 6 credits. If a worker becomes disabled before age 24, the worker is specially insured for disability benefits if he or she has 6 quarters of credit in the 12 quarter period immediately prior to becoming disabled.

Determining Disability

The Social Security Administration will only determine an eligible worker to be disabled when he or she lacks the ability to do any substantial gainful activity by reason of any medically determinable physical or mental impairment that can be expected to result in death or which has lasted (or can be expected to last) for a continuous period of not less than twelve months. The impairment must be so severe that the worker must be unable to do his or her previous work or any other substantial gainful activity which exists in the national economy. The Social Security Disability Insurance monthly payment is based on the worker's past earnings. There is usually a five-month waiting period before these payments begin.

Working While Receiving Disability Benefits

"Substantial gainful activity" (SGA) is the ability to perform work that produces earnings. Beginning in 2015, earnings of $1,090 per month or more is considered substantial. If a worker's earnings average less than $1,090 per month, the worker's disability benefits should continue. For a blind person, earnings of $1,820 or more will be considered substantial in the year 2015.

Disabled Widow's/Widower's Benefits

A disabled widow or widower of a deceased worker is entitled to receive Social Security if he or she is between the ages of 50 and 60. A subsequent marriage after age 50 will not affect the right to receive social security as the disabled widow or widower of a deceased spouse. Should the disabled widow or widower who remarried before age 50 divorce the new spouse or should the new spouse die, the death or divorce would re-establish the disabled widow's or widower's eligibility to benefits. If a disabled spouse is eligible for multiple benefits as a widow or widower of several spouses, he or she has the option of taking the highest monthly benefit.

Family Benefits for a Disabled Worker

A spouse and each dependent child of a disabled worker will also be eligible for a monthly Social Security benefit. When combined, these family benefits cannot exceed 150 percent of the disabled worker's retirement benefit.

CHAPTER 2

MEDICARE

- Medicare Part A
  - Hospital Care
  - Skilled Nursing Facility Care
  - Home Health Care
  - Hospice
- Medicare Part B
- Qualified Medicare Beneficiary
- Specified Low Income Medicare Beneficiary
- Medigap Insurance Policy
- Medicare Advantage
- Medicare Part D

Congress approved Medicare in 1965 to pay some of the cost of health care services for the aged. In order to receive this assistance with the current cost of health care, a person must be 65 years of age or older and entitled to Social Security retirement insurance or Railroad Retirement cash benefits. A person who has received Social Security disability benefits or Railroad Retirement Disability Income for 24 months or longer is also entitled to receive Medicare assistance regardless of his or her age. However, an application to enroll in Medicare must be filed by this disabled person. An application for Medicare can be filed after receiving 21 months of disability benefits. Persons of any age who have end-stage renal disease or amyotrophic lateral sclerosis can also apply for this coverage.

There are three basic threshold criteria for Medicare coverage:
1. The care and supplies to be provided must be medically reasonable and necessary for diagnosis or treatment of illness or injury or to improve the functioning of a malformed body part.
2. The care and supplies must be prescribed by a doctor.
3. The services and the supplies must be obtained through a Medicare-certified provider.

Medicare seldom pays all the costs of health care. In many areas of coverage, the patient is required to pay a specified deductible amount each year or during each illness. In addition, the patient may have to pay for a portion of the cost. Medicare calls this a co-insurance payment or co-payment.

The present Medicare program provides two separate packages of benefits, Part A and Part B. A person who is 65 years of age and who is entitled to Social Security or Railroad Retirement benefits is automatically enrolled in Medicare Part A and will be deemed to have enrolled in Medicare Part B. A person who is not receiving Social Security or Railroad Retirement Benefits must enroll for Medicare Part A during the initial enrollment period. This period begins in the third month before the person attains age 65 and extends for the next seven months. A person who takes early Social Security retirement is automatically enrolled in Medicare when he or she attains age 65.

A person aged 65 and older (or a person under age 65 who is disabled) who has not received credit from Social Security for 40 quarters of coverage may enroll in Medicare Part A, but he or she may have to pay a $407 per month premium in 2015 if the individual has 29 or fewer quarters of Social Security credits. Eligible individuals with 30-39 quarters of Social Security credits must pay a $234 per month premium in 2015.

Medicare Part A

Medicare Part A covers acute hospital care, a limited number of skilled nursing facility days, home health care and hospice care.

Hospital Care

Hospital coverage is available when the care and treatment needed can only be rendered on an inpatient basis at a hospital or a critical access hospital. Hospital coverage can be extended if a patient who would otherwise be discharged requires a skilled nursing facility level of care and no appropriate placement in a Medicare-certified skilled nursing facility is available.

The spell of illness concept is central to coverage for hospital and skilled nursing facility care. A spell of illness begins on the day a patient first receives inpatient care. It ends when a Medicare beneficiary has not been in a hospital or skilled nursing facility as an inpatient for 60 consecutive days, or has not received a Medicare-covered level of care for 60 days. There can be more than one spell of illness in a given calendar year. This will give rise to a second deductible, new co-insurance amounts and a new set of hospital days.

Medicare Part A will pay for inpatient hospital care that is medically necessary for treatment or diagnosis after the patient meets the initial first day deductible, which is $1,260 in 2015. Benefits cover 90 days of inpatient hospital care for each spell of illness. There is a $315 per day deductible for the 61st through 90th day in the hospital during the same spell of illness in 2015. In addition, a patient is allowed a maximum of 60 lifetime reserve days with a $630 per day deductible in 2015. Each year, there is an adjustment to the initial deductible, co-insurance amount and lifetime reserve daily amount. This adjustment is normally published in October of the year preceding the new calendar year in which the new deductible will apply.

Maximum Coverage for Hospital Care (2015)

Days in Hospital	How Much You Pay	How Much Medicare Pays
First 60 days	$1,260 for first day	Balance
61-90 days	$315/day	Balance
91-150 days	$630/day	Balance
After 150 days	All Costs	Nothing

Medicare covers a lifetime maximum of 190 days of inpatient psychiatric hospital care. This is in addition to the coverage for hospital care described above. However, a person can only use 150 of these days for this care in one benefit period. Also, this care is subject to the same deductibles and co-insurance, which is described above for other forms of hospitalization.

Coverage under Part A includes the hospital room on a semiprivate basis, nursing services, operating room costs, prescriptions and medical supplies, laboratory tests and x-rays provided by the hospital as part of its services. While in a hospital, physician services are not covered under Part A. The physician services provided while in a hospital will be billed under Medicare Part B. Certain luxury items (private rooms, private duty nurses, television, and telephone) are not covered by Medicare. Medicare does not pay for the first three units of blood that are received in a hospital in any calendar year. This blood deductible is in addition to the deductibles and co-insurance described above. However, the Part B blood deductible may apply.

LIFE SITUATION #4

Joseph, who is over 65, was hospitalized for 20 days, received 30 days of skilled care in a nursing facility, and went home for 62 days before being readmitted to a hospital. The first "spell of illness" ended 60 days after the expiration of Joseph's stay in the nursing facility. A new spell of illness will be triggered by the second hospitalization. New inpatient hospital deductibles must be paid.

Skilled Nursing Facility Care

There are many restrictions that apply to Medicare coverage for skilled nursing facility care. Skilled nursing care requires that the care must be provided by or requires the supervision of skilled nursing personnel or other skilled rehabilitation services, which as a practical matter can only be provided in a skilled nursing home facility on an inpatient basis. Medicare never extends coverage to a patient who needs custodial care only. For each spell of illness, Medicare Part A will pay all the costs for a covered skilled nursing home stay for the first 20 days and all but $157.50 per day in 2015 for up to an additional 80 days as long as all of the following conditions are met:

1. The individual was a patient in a hospital for three consecutive days not including the day of discharge. In addition, the patient must be admitted to the skilled nursing facility within 30 days of discharge from the hospital. (Note: there are a few limited exceptions to the requirement that the admission must occur within 30 days of discharge from the hospital).
2. A doctor must certify that the patient needs skilled nursing home care.
3. The services the patient needs must include either daily skilled nursing or skilled rehabilitation services (or a combination of these services).
4. The services are provided by or under the supervision of a trained individual.
5. The services are received on a daily basis, which means therapy services at least 5 days per week and/or nursing care 7 days per week.
6. The services are provided by a Medicare-certified skilled nursing facility.
7. The skilled services must be provided on an inpatient basis.

A Medicare beneficiary is entitled to receive coverage for skilled care in a nursing home (subject to the following co-payments in 2014):

Days in SNF	How much you pay	How much Medicare Pays
First 20 days	Nothing	100 percent of approved amount
Additional 80 days	$157.50/day	Balance
Beyond 100	All Costs	Nothing

Home Health Care

A Medicare home health benefit can be available under Medicare Part A or Medicare Part B. However, Medicare Part A home health care benefits are limited to 100 visits and must follow a prior hospital or skilled nursing facility stay. The threshold criteria for home health care is as follows:

1. The patient must be generally confined to the home. This means that this individual's condition must be such that the patient requires assistance to leave home (such as crutches, cane, walker, or assistance of another person, etc.) or that leaving the home without assistance is not advisable, and that leaving home requires a considerable effort. This is often known as the homebound requirement.
2. The home health care must be included in a plan of care by a doctor.
3. The patient must require skilled care. This means speech or physical therapy service or intermittent skilled nursing care. Occupational therapy will count toward the required skilled care, if it had been originally provided in conjunction with physical therapy, speech therapy, or skilled nursing.
4. The services rendered must be medically reasonable and necessary.
5. The services must be provided by, or under arrangements with, a Medicare certified home health agency.

Once these criteria have all been met, several medical services are fully paid for by Medicare, including the following:

1. Part-time or intermittent nursing care provided by or under the supervision of a registered professional nurse.
2. Physical, occupational, and speech therapy.
3. Medical social services under the direction of a physician.
4. Part-time home health aide services.

Until now, Medicare providers were required to use an "improvement standard" in determining whether Medicare will pay for therapy requiring ~~skilled~~ care. Thus, Medicare beneficiaries were denied skilled care coverage if the therapy will not restore or improve the beneficiary's health or physical condition. This meant that Medicare beneficiaries were denied coverage by Medicare for skilled therapies that are only necessary to maintain the patient's current condition or to prevent or slow further deterioration.

On January 24, 2013, the U.S. District Court for Vermont approved a Settlement Agreement involving the Center For Medicare and Medicaid Services that states Medicare will now also provide reimbursement for skilled therapies necessary to maintain the patient's current condition or to prevent or slow further deterioration. The case is entitled Jimmo v. Sebelius, 2011 WL 5104355 (D. Vermont) Jan. 25, 2013). The case clarifies that the standard for determining Medicare coverage for skilled care will also include those services that are necessary to maintain the patient's current physical condition or to prevent or slow further deterioration. This is known as the maintenance coverage standard. To be considered a skilled service, the service must be so inherently complex that it can be safely and effectively performed only by, or under the supervision of, professional or technical personnel.

It is important to understand that this new standard for Medicare coverage of skilled maintenance services applies now to Medicare recipients throughout the entire United States of America.

Hospice

To be entitled to Medicare hospice coverage, a person must be certified as terminally ill. This means that a physician must state that in his or her clinical judgment, the person's life expectancy is six months or less if the illness follows its expected course. In addition, the patient must waive all rights to Medicare payments for the duration of the hospice care for any regular Medicare services related treatment of the terminal illness. Instead, the patient elects to receive palliative services provided under the arrangement of the hospice or provided by an attending physician, if the attending physician is not an employee of the hospice.

The primary advantage of hospice Medicare is that a terminal patient's broad needs can be met with a hidden array of services for a longer period of time. Hospice care provides the terminally ill patient with a holistic approach that concentrates on the patient's pain management, offers specialized care, and attempts to meet the spiritual and emotional needs of the patient and his or her family. The hospice patient is liable for co-insurance amounts only for respite care and drugs. However, the co-insurance cannot exceed $5 per prescription. It is important to remember that only medications for palliative purposes are covered under the hospice benefit.

Medicare hospice is often more economical to the patient and the patient's family than hospital, home health, and nursing home care. This is because the increased care allowed the hospice patient is provided regardless of the patient's ability to pay. For instance, the hospice provider pays for all of the cost of the hospice patient's prescriptions that are necessary for the patient's control of the pain at home and the related symptoms associated with the terminal illness. However, in some instances, the regular home health benefit may provide equal or better coverage.

Medicare hospice provides physician services, nursing services, social services, counseling services to the terminally ill and family members, short-term inpatient care provided in a hospice inpatient unit or in a hospital or skilled nursing facility, medical appliances and supplies, drugs, home health aid services, homemaker services and physical therapy provided for symptom control or to help the patient maintain activities of daily living.

The hospice benefit is divided into periods. The first two benefit periods are 90 days, followed by an unlimited number of 60-day periods. A person may designate another hospice one time in each election period.

In addition, a person may opt out of, and return to, Medicare hospice coverage at any time. Medicare Part A coverage that was waived when the Medicare hospice benefit was elected is automatically resumed with the effective cancellation date. To opt back into hospice, a new election form and physicians certificate is necessary.

It is important to remember that Medicare Advantage plans may provide, but are not required to provide, hospice care to their beneficiaries. A beneficiary may change the designation of the particular hospice from which the care will be received once each election period.

Medicare Part B

Medicare Part B is a voluntary program for persons who are 65 years of age or older who are citizens or who have been a lawful permanent resident for five years preceding the date of the application. The major benefit under Medicare Part B is payment of the physician's charges for surgery, consultations, office visits and the physician's visits to the patient's hospital or nursing home room. Durable medical equipment, outpatient physical therapy, X-rays, and diagnostic tests are also covered. Medicare Part B also covers home health visits not covered under Part A.

Medicare Part B does not cover prescription drugs that do not require administration by a physician, routine physical checkups, eyeglasses, eye exams to prescribe eyeglasses, hearing aids or hearing exams for hearing aids, dental services and routine foot care. Ambulance transportation is only covered when other modes of transportation would be harmful to the patient. For a non-emergency trip to be covered, the patient must not be able to rise out of bed without assistance, be unable to walk and unable to sit in a chair or wheelchair. Ambulance service that is not an emergency must be certified in advance with a doctor's written order certifying that the patient meets these criteria.

Preventive care services, checkups and comfort items are for the most part not covered under Medicare. However, certain preventative care services are now covered under Medicare Part B due to laws being passed that specifically include these services. These services include, for Medicare eligible persons, an annual mammogram for women enrolled who are age 40 and older, Pap smears and pelvic exams for beneficiaries considered a high risk following an abnormal Pap smear. A woman not in this group is entitled to a Pap smear and a pelvic exam once every two years. The deductible does not apply to these procedures. Prostate screening for men over age 50 and colorectal cancer screening tests for beneficiaries age 50 or older are also included.

A person who is enrolled under Medicare Part A is assumed to want coverage under Medicare Part B. A person covered under Medicare Part A may decline to be covered under Medicare Part B before the coverage begins or within 2 months after being notified that Medicare Part B coverage has commenced.

Medicare Part B has an annual deductible requirement of at least $147 in 2015. Each year, before Medicare pays anything, the patient must incur medical expenses equal to the deductible, based on Medicare's approved reasonable charge, not on the provider's actual charge. In addition, there is a co-insurance amount which the patient must pay. This is equal to 20 percent of the Medicare approved amount.

Most Medicare beneficiaries will pay a $104.90 Part B premium amount each month in 2015. However, there is a Part B premium surcharge for high income individuals and married couples that is based on that person's or couple's 2012 adjusted gross income plus tax-exempt income. An individual who in 2013 had annual income greater than $85,000 and married couples who had income in 2013 greater than $170,000 will pay a Part B Medicare premium of $146.90 per month in 2015. An individual with income for 2013 greater than $107,000 and married couples with 2013 income greater than $214,000 will pay a monthly premium of $209.80 in 2014. An individual with annual income in 2013 greater than $160,000 and married couples with an annual income in 2013 greater than $320,000 will pay a monthly premium in 2015 of $272.70 each. Individuals with annual incomes greater than $214,000 and married couples with annual incomes greater than $428,000 in 2013 will pay a monthly premium of $335.70 per month in 2015. Income is calculated by taking a beneficiary's adjusted gross income and adding back in some normally excluded income, such as tax-exempt interest, U.S. savings bond interest used to pay tuition, and certain income from foreign sources. This is called modified adjusted gross income (MAGI). If a beneficiary's MAGI decreased significantly in the past two years, he or she may request that information from more recent years be used to calculate the premium.

A major problem with Medicare Part B is the difference between the cost of medical items or services, particularly physician's services, and the Medicare-approved reasonable charge. When an item or service is determined to be covered under Medicare, it is reimbursed at 80 percent of the reasonable charge for the item or service, and the patient is responsible for the remaining 20 percent. Unfortunately, the reasonable charge set by Medicare may often be substantially less than the actual charge. The result of the reasonable-charge reimbursement system is that the Medicare payment, even for items and services covered by Part B, is often insufficient to pay the complete amount of the charge for the service. The patient is thus left with out-of-pocket expenses. However, when a physician accepts Medicare assignment, he or she agrees to accept the Medicare-approved amount as full payment. Medicare will pay 80 percent and the patient is responsible to pay the 20 percent co-payment. When a physician does not accept assignment, the patient is liable for the co-payment plus a balance above the Medicare fee schedule amount. However, under federal law, there is a set limit (limiting charge) that the physician may charge. A physician not accepting assignment for payment of a Medicare claim may submit a balanced bill that does not exceed 115 percent of the Medicare-approved amount. The patient's Medicare Summary Notice will state the Medicare approved charge for the doctor's services.

LIFE SITUATION #5
Mary is treated by a doctor who does not accept Medicare assignment. This physician's actual charge is $100, but the Medicare fee schedule states the allowable charge is only $70. This doctor may charge Mary only 115 percent of the scheduled amount, or $80.50, for this service, since the doctor has not agreed to accept assignment of the Medicare benefit. Mary would be responsible for paying the physician the entire $80.50 and then requesting Medicare to reimburse her $56 ($70 x 80 percent). If the doctor accepted assignment, the doctor would file Mary's claim and request her to pay $14 ($70 x 20%).

Qualified Medicare Beneficiary

A person 65 years of age or older or a disabled individual receiving Medicare may qualify for assistance with the payment of Medicare deductibles. Florida's Children and Families' Medicaid Department will pay this beneficiary's Medicare Part B premium and co-insurance and the Medicare Part A deductibles if this individual has income at or lower than $990 per month. A married couple has the same entitlement if their combined income is lower than $1,335 per month. These income caps may increase when published for 2015. In addition, the beneficiary's countable assets must be less than $7,160 and a married couple's countable assets may not exceed $10,750. Non-countable assets are the homestead, one car, a burial plot, $2,500 deposited in a burial savings account and life insurance policies having a total face value of less than $2,500.

Specified Low Income Medicare Beneficiary

A Specified Low Income Medicare Beneficiary is a person 65 years of age or older or a disabled individual receiving Medicare who has income at or lower than $1,187 per month or a couple with income lower than $1,602 per month. These income caps may increase when published for 2015. In addition, the beneficiary's countable assets must be less than $7,160 and a married couple's assets may not exceed $10,750. Only the Specified Low Income Medicare Beneficiary's Part B premium is paid by Florida's Children and Families' Medicaid Department. The Medicare Part A deductible and the Medicare Part A co-insurance must still be paid by this Medicare beneficiary.

Medigap Insurance Policy

"Medigap" is the term used to describe the supplemental insurance policy needed to cover the health care costs, deductibles and co-pay amounts not provided by Medicare. This policy is important for Medicare recipients who rely on traditional Medicare coverage Medicare Part A.

The standardized Medigap policies that may be sold are as follows:

Plan A contains the basic or "core" benefits. The following is a list of the benefits that are contained in the core policy and that must be contained in all Medigap policies:

1.   Part A hospital co-insurance for days 61 to 90 ($315 per day in the year 2015);
2.   Part A lifetime reserve co-insurance for days 91 to 150 ($630 in 2015);
3.   Part B 20% co-insurance or co-payment;
4.   365 lifetime hospital days beyond Medicare coverage;
5.   Hospice Care co-payment;
6.   Parts A and B three pint blood deductible;

The other Medigap policies contain the core benefits plus one or more additional benefits are as follows:

- Plan B policies contain the core coverage and 100% of the Part A deductible.
- Plan C policies contain the core coverage; the skilled nursing home facility co-insurance, 100% of the Part A and Part B deductibles, and foreign travel care.
- Plan D policies contain the core coverage plus 100% of the Part A deductible, SNF co-insurance, and 80% of foreign travel care.
- Plan E is no longer available since it included the same coverage as plan D.
- Plan F contains the core coverage plus 100% of the Part A and Part B deductible, SNF benefits plus; 100% of Part B excess charges; and 80% of foreign travel care. However, there is a $2,180 Medicare deductible in 2015 that is adjusted each year.
- Plan G contains the core coverage plus 100% of the Part A deductible, 50% of the Part B deductible, 50% of the SNF benefits and 80% of foreign travel care.
- Plan H has been discontinued since it provided the same coverage as plan D but with drug coverage that is no longer necessary due to Medicare Part D.
- Plan I has been discontinued since it provided the same coverage as plan G but with drug coverage that is no longer necessary due to Medicare Part D.

- Plan J has been discontinued since it provided the same coverage as plan F but with drug coverage that is no longer necessary due to Medicare Part D.
- Plan K contains the core coverage plus 100% of Part A deductible plus 50% of the Part B deductible: 50% of Hospice care, 50% of reasonable cost for three pints of blood plus 50% of the Part A deductible.
- Plan L contains the core coverage and 100% of the Part A hospital co-insurance plus 75% of the Part B deductible: 75% of Hospice care, 75% of reasonable cost for three pints of blood plus 75% of the Part A deductible.
- Plan M contains the core benefits plus 50% of the Part A deductible, the skilled nursing facility co-insurance, plus 50% of the Part A deductible and 80% of the foreign travel care.
- Plan N contains the core benefits plus 100% of the Part A deductible, the skilled nursing facility co-insurance, and 80% of the foreign travel care and the lesser of $20 or the Part B co-insurance/co-payment for office visit (including specialists) and the lesser of $50 or Part B co-insurance/co-payment for emergency room visits. The co-payment waived if patient admitted to hospital and the emergency visit is subsequently covered under Part A.

Medicare Advantage

The ever increasing cost of the Medicare deductibles, the Medicare supplement and the additional cost of the Medicare Part D prescription drug plan will eventually drive most of the 35 million fee-for-service Medicare beneficiaries into joining the 15.7 million Medicare beneficiaries presently enrolled in a Medicare Advantage plan. These services are found in Part C of the Medicare Statutes. This is known as a Medicare Advantage plan. A Medicare Advantage plan is owned by a private company that provides all of a beneficiary's health care and prescriptions through the plan's health care providers for a capitated rate paid by the Centers for Medicare and Medicaid. The Medicare Advantage company must provide all the services currently available under Medicare Parts A and B. The primary physician who is assigned to the Medicare Advantage beneficiary serves as a gatekeeper to specialists. Thus, the beneficiary's health care cost is reduced while his or her health is maintained. However, a Medicare Advantage beneficiary loses the right to select any doctor and must select from a panel of physicians offered by the plan.

Every year in November, the Center for Medicare and Medicaid conducts an annual coordinated enrollment period during which time all Medicare beneficiaries are able to choose between the original Medicare program and a Medicare Advantage plan. A Medicare beneficiary has between October 15 and December 7 to join, switch or drop a Medicare

Advantage Plan. The coverage begins on January 1 of the ensuing year, as long as the plan receives the request by December 7th. Between January 1 – 14, a person who is a member of a Medicare Advantage Plan can leave his or her plan and switch to the original Medicare. If a person switches to the original Medicare during this period, he or she will have until February 14 to also select a Medicare Prescription Drug Plan to add drug coverage. The coverage will begin the first day of the month after the enrollment form is received. Although Medicare Advantage may seem to save beneficiaries more money at first, they will only save money if the Medicare beneficiary uses the plan's doctors for all their care. In addition, because Medicare Advantage plans only have one-year contracts, the provider can decide to change its costs and even leave the Medicare program.

Medicare Part D

Medicare's prescription drug program began on January 1, 2006. This program known as Medicare Part D provides limited financial assistance with drug expenses to persons enrolled under Medicare Part A or Part B who pay the additional Part D premium to a private company. These prescription drug plans offered pursuant to Medicare Part D are provided by private companies. Thus, a person eligible for Medicare must affirmatively enroll in a voluntary prescription drug coverage program under Medicare Part D for one year at a time. Medicare Advantage Plans normally provide prescription coverage.

It is important to understand that the drugs offered by different plans vary. This new law does not authorize the establishment of specific lists of medications that must be offered by the Medicare Part D formularies. In general, once a person selects a prescription drug plan, he or she is locked in to the drug plan and cannot change until the next annual enrollment period. This is true even though the plan in which he or she enrolls changes the formulary or cost sharing arrangement, with enrollment in the new plan becoming effective January 1 of the following year. The annual enrollment period for Medicare Part D is between October 15th and December 7th of each year. During this period, a person who is eligible for Medicare can enroll in a plan or change his or her enrollment from one plan to another. An individual who is already in a plan can decide if he or she wants to remain in the same plan for the current year or if he or she wants to select another plan. There is a late penalty for failure to timely enroll when a person is first eligible. The penalty is 1% of the national average premium for every month that a person delays enrollment. Thus, a person who becomes eligible to enroll in Part D at age 65 and delays enrolling until age 66 can be assessed a 12% penalty on his or her premium for the remainder of his or her life. The amount of the penalty will vary each year as the national average premium changes. However, this penalty is waived if a person had creditable coverage with an employer or through the Veterans Administration or Tricare. Creditable coverage means that the employer's drug plan is equivalent to the Part D benefit.

The monthly premium that a Medicare beneficiary will have to pay on a monthly basis for Part D drug benefits varies from company to company and depends on the formulary being provided by that company. However, the monthly premium will be more if your income reported to the IRS two years ago was more than $85,000. The Part D premium surcharge for high income individuals and married couples that is based on that person's or couple's 2013 adjusted gross income plus tax-exempt income. An individual who in 2013 had annual income greater than $85,000 and married couples who had income in 2013 greater than $170,000 will pay a monthly premium of $12.30 plus his or her plan premium per month in 2015. An individual with income for 2013 greater than $107,000 and married couples with 2013 income greater than $214,000 will pay a monthly premium of $31.80 plus his or her monthly plan premium in 2015. An individual with annual income in 2013 greater than $160,000 and married couples with an annual income in 2013 greater than $320,000 will pay a monthly premium in 2015 of $51.30 plus the plan premium. Individuals with annual incomes greater than $214,000 and married couples with annual incomes greater than $428,000 in 2013 will pay a monthly premium of $71.80 plus his or her plan premium.

A Medicare beneficiary who elects to pay this premium will then pay an annual deductible for prescriptions. The average Medicare Part D premium costs are expected to be around $31 per month. The annual deductible for 2015 will vary by plan. However, the maximum annual deductible for 2015 cannot exceed the first $325 of prescription drug expenses incurred during 2015 for drugs on the plan's list of covered drugs or formulary. The enrolled Medicare beneficiary then pays a co-insurance amount of his or her 2015 prescription costs, for formulary drugs, in excess of the annual deductible up to the initial coverage limit in 2015 of $2,960. The Medicare beneficiary's prescription drug plan sponsor pays the remaining cost. The Medicare beneficiary then enters the Donut Hole. The Affordable Care Act then provides that the drug manufacturer will discount 35% of the cost of generic drugs and 55% of the cost of the brand-name drugs while you are in what is called the donut hole. Once you have paid an additional $3,720 in prescription drug costs for 2015, you will have reached what is called the catastrophic coverage limit of the Medicare Part D Program. You will then only have to pay a co-payment of $2.55 for a generic drug and $6.50 for all other drugs.

The annual premium and the deductibles are expected to increase each year as the cost of this additional Medicare benefit increases. Prescription costs will be treated as incurred by the Medicare beneficiary only if they are paid by the eligible beneficiary or by another individual on behalf of the eligible beneficiary. If the eligible individual is reimbursed for such costs through insurance, a group health plan, or other third-party payment arrangement, the prescription cost may not count toward the eligible beneficiary's incurred share of cost.

A Medicare beneficiary can only make changes to his or her Part D coverage for 2015 during the Annual Enrollment Period which is between October 15 and December 7 of 2014. Thus, a Medicare beneficiary who is not satisfied with his or her Medicare Part D provider during 2015, should note his or her calendar to change to another plan after October 15th, but before December 7th of the year 2015.

CHAPTER 3

TAXATION OF PENSION PLAN AND IRA DISTRIBUTIONS

- Distribution of Pension Plan Benefits
- Premature Distributions
- Required Distributions
- Distributions During the Participant's Lifetime
- Distributions Upon Participant's Death Before Required Beginning Date
- Distributions Upon Participant's Death After Required Date
- Rollover by Surviving Spouse
- Inherited IRA
- Trust as Beneficiary
- Roth IRA
- IRA Contribution Limits
- Estate Taxation of IRA Distributions

Distribution of Pension Plan Benefits

Distribution from a pension plan must commence within 60 days after the end of the plan year in which the participant attains normal retirement age unless the participant continues to work for the employer or does not have 10 years of vested service. The normal retirement age for the participant of a qualified pension plan is the earlier of the age that the plan provides for normal retirement or the date that the plan participant attains age 65. An exception exists for a plan participant who commenced participation in the pension plan within 5 years before attaining normal retirement age under the plan. In that instance, normal retirement age is the fifth anniversary date from the date the participant commenced participation in the plan.

A pension plan must state that a vested employee who retires will receive the benefit in the form of a qualified joint and survivor annuity, unless the participant and his or her spouse elect otherwise. This means that if the participant dies, the surviving spouse will continue to receive no less than 50 percent of the monthly benefit payable to the participant.

Since the distribution from a pension plan will be subject to ordinary income tax in the year received, a retired beneficiary of a pension plan may want to defer the taxation of these distributions by electing to rollover these benefits into an Individual Retirement Account (IRA) within 60 days of distribution of the plan benefits.

29

Premature Distributions

A premature distribution will occur when a participant in a retirement plan or an owner of an Individual Retirement Account (IRA) receives a distribution of money from the retirement plan or IRA before the age of 59 and a half years. The IRS penalizes a premature distribution with an additional 10 percent excise tax except in the following circumstances:

1. The distribution is made to a beneficiary of the IRA or pension plan (or to the participant's estate) upon the death of the participant.

2. The distribution is made to a participant who has become disabled and can no longer engage in substantial gainful activity.

3. The distributions are paid to the participant of a pension plan at least annually in substantially equal installments over the life expectancy of the participant or the joint life expectancy of the participant and the participant's beneficiary. This distribution provision is available to a participant at any age.

4. The distributions the participant receives from a pension plan are used to pay his or her medical expenses that exceed 7.5 percent of the participant's adjusted gross income.

5. The distribution represents an interest in a pension plan that is paid as a result of a divorce decree and pursuant to a Qualified Domestic Retirement Order.

6. The pension plan distribution is to a person who is at least 55 years of age and is receiving the distribution as a result of separation from service.

7. The IRA distribution is to a person who uses up to $10,000 of the proceeds to buy his or her first residence or the first residence of his or her spouse, child, grand child or ancestor or the account holder's spouse.

8. The IRA distribution is for educational expenses incurred by the taxpayer, his or her spouse, or the children or grandchildren of either the taxpayer or his or her spouse. This law applies only to distributions from IRAs and not to those from employer pension plans.

9. The distribution is rolled into an IRA or another qualified retirement plan within 60 days of receipt.

10. Withdrawals from an IRA are used by the account holder to pay for medical insurance for the account holder and the account holders spouse and dependents if the account holder has received unemployment compensation for 12 consecutive weeks under any federal or state unemployment compensation law.

11. The distribution is made on account of a federal tax levy.

Required Distributions

A participant of a pension plan or an owner of a traditional IRA must begin receiving minimum distributions from a qualified pension plan or traditional IRA by the time he or she reaches the required beginning date. The required beginning date is the first day of April of the calendar year following the calendar year in which the participant or owner is age 70 1/2. It is important to remember that waiting until the required beginning date to receive the first distribution will require the participant to receive the second annual distribution by December 31 of the same year to meet the minimum distribution rules. The two distributions in one year could place the participant in a higher tax bracket for that year.

The Internal Revenue Code extends the required beginning date for a participant of a pension plan who remains an employee to the first day of April of the year following the year in which an employee retires. This exception applies only if the participant continues to work beyond the age of 70 ½ and does not own more than 5 percent of the stock of the company where he or she continues to work. If an employee owns 5 percent of the company from 65 to 70 1/2, he or she will be deemed to be a 5 percent owner as of age 70 1/2. Since the Internal Revenue Service has not defined retirement for the purpose of this code section, it is uncertain whether this exception will apply to a person who continues to work only part-time.

It is important to remember that an excise tax is imposed if the amount distributed from a retirement plan or IRA is less than the required minimum distribution. This excise tax is 50 percent of the amount that should have been distributed in a year minus the amount actually distributed that year.

The Internal Revenue Service regulations relating to the required minimum distributions apply to pension plans, individual retirement accounts (but not Roth IRAs), profit sharing plans, section 401(k) plans, section 403(b) plans and any other deferred income benefits that have not been subject to income tax and which will become taxable income when received. The mortality tables have been modified to reflect current life expectancy. The new tables are used to determine an employee's or IRA owner's life expectancy under the single life table and the uniform lifetime table. New tables are also used to determine the joint life and last survivor expectancy of an employee or IRA owner and the designated beneficiary.

IRA trustees, custodians, and issuers must provide information relating to lifetime required minimum distributions to IRA owners by January 31. The IRA trustee must either provide the IRA owner with the amount of the required minimum distribution for that year, or offer to provide the IRA owner, upon request, with the amount of the required minimum distribution for that year. The fact that a minimum distribution is required with respect to an IRA for a year must be reported by the IRA trustee to the IRS. However, the trustee does not report the amount of the required minimum distribution.

Distributions During the Participant's Lifetime

The minimum distribution rules provide for the use of a simple, uniform lifetime table that all employees or IRA owners can use to determine the minimum distribution required during their lifetime. The distribution table assumes a continuing life expectancy of 27.4 years for an individual 70 years old. The only exception to the use of this uniform minimum distribution period table is when the designated beneficiary has a spouse more than 10 years younger than the IRA owner. In this instance, a separate joint and survivor expectancy table must be used to determine the required annual minimum distribution.

The marital status is determined at the beginning of the year. Since the annual distribution schedule starts at about 4 percent, an IRA owner earning 5 percent each year will accumulate excess income between ages 71 and age 80. It is only in later years that the minimum annual pay out increases to the point that all of the annual income and some of the principal must be distributed. This means that there will often be a balance left when the IRA owner dies.

Distributions Upon Participant's Death
Before Required Beginning Date

If a participant dies before reaching his or her required beginning date and he or she has designated a beneficiary, his or her plan benefits and IRA proceeds will be distributed over the designated beneficiary's life expectancy, beginning no later than the end of the calendar year in which the participant died. If the participant's sole designated beneficiary is his or her surviving spouse, the distribution must commence by the end of the calendar year in which the participant would have attained age 70 1/2. If not, it must be rolled over and distributions must commence by December 31 of the calendar year following the calendar year in which the spouse attained age 70 1/2. If there is no designated beneficiary and the owner dies before his or her required beginning date, the distributions must be made within five (5) years after the deceased owner's death.

Distributions Upon Participant's Death
After Required Beginning Date

If a participant dies after reaching his or her required beginning date, the distribution can be over the life expectancy of the beneficiary or the life expectancy of the deceased. If there is no designated beneficiary, then the distribution must be over no more than 5 years after the date of the death of the participant. However, if the sole designated beneficiary is the spouse, the applicable distribution period is the spouse's life expectancy determined each year until his or her death, at which point it becomes the life expectancy of the spouse determined in the calendar year of the spouse's death, reduced by one for each calendar year that has elapsed since the calendar year immediately following the year of the spouse's death.

Rollover by Surviving Spouse

A surviving spouse of a deceased participant or IRA owner has the right to rollover the plan benefits or IRA proceeds into his or her IRA, or to treat the deceased spouse's IRA as his or her own. The surviving spouse will be treated as the participant's sole designated beneficiary to the extent he or she is the outright designated beneficiary of some or all of the participant's plan benefit or IRA. If the spouse is the designated beneficiary and decides not to roll the IRA over into his or her name, distributions to the surviving spouse must be paid over the remaining life expectancy of the surviving spouse. However, the beginning date for these distributions may be deferred until the latter of the calendar year following the year in which the employee died, or the end of the calendar year in which the employee would have attained age 70 and one half.

If the plan benefit or IRA is payable to more than one beneficiary, and the surviving spouse is one of those beneficiaries, he or she will not be treated as the surviving spouse's sole beneficiary unless, by September 30 of the calendar year following the calendar year of the participant's death, the other beneficiaries have been cashed out, have disclaimed their right to receive the plan benefit or IRA, or a separate account has been created for the portion of the plan benefit or IRA to which the surviving spouse is entitled. While a disclaimer can be given at any time before the beneficiary determination date, it is important to remember that it will not be a qualified disclaimer unless it is given within nine months of death. Otherwise, the disclaimer will result in the disclaiming beneficiary having made a taxable gift.

Inherited IRA

Prior to the year 2007, if the IRA owner died before distributions began, the entire IRA had to be distributed by December 31 of the fifth year following the year of the owner's death, unless the beneficiary was the surviving spouse. The law now permits the beneficiary to exclude all the proceeds from becoming immediately taxable by transferring the account to a new separate inherited IRA that is opened in the name of the deceased to receive the proceeds. The new IRA must be designated as an inherited IRA. The new account must name the same persons as the beneficiaries. Although the beneficiaries now own the IRA, the IRA is not titled in the beneficiary's name. In addition, the beneficiary cannot contribute to this new account. A suggested way of titling the account would be, "Harry Jones, deceased, for the benefit of Richard Jones, beneficiary." The advantage of an Inherited IRA is that the beneficiary generally will not owe tax on the assets in the Inherited IRA until the beneficiary receives distributions from it which will be over a period not extending beyond the life expectancy of the designated beneficiary. The beneficiary must choose which rule is to apply by December 31 of the year following the year of the owner's death. This is because a distribution generally must begin under the life expectancy rule. If no decision is timely made, then distribution will be made over the beneficiary's life expectancy.

If there is more than one beneficiary as of the end of the year following the year in which the owner dies, the beneficiary with the shortest life expectancy will be the designated beneficiary if all of the beneficiaries are individuals, and the account or benefit has not been divided into separate accounts or shares for each beneficiary.

In the recent case of Clark v. Rameker, the Supreme Court of the United States ruled on whether the beneficiary of an inherited IRA in Wisconsin could claim an exemption from the claims of creditors under the federal Bankruptcy Code. In Clark, Ruth Heffron had owned a traditional IRA and named her daughter, Heidi Heffron-Clark, as the sole beneficiary. When Ruth Heffron died, her IRA passed to her daughter as an inherited IRA. The daughter, Heidi Heffron-Clark, later petitioned for Chapter 7 bankruptcy and claimed that the monies in her inherited IRA were exempt "retirement funds" the Bankruptcy Code.

The bankruptcy trustee objected and the Bankruptcy Court agreed, refusing to allow the exemption. The District Court reversed, reasoning that the exemption covers any funds originally accumulated for retirement purposes. The Seventh Circuit reversed the District Court on the grounds that inherited IRAs allow for current consumption and are not designed as a fund for retirement savings. Accordingly, the issue in the case was whether inherited IRAs meet the definition of "retirement funds" in order to receive creditor protection in bankruptcy.

In general, section 522 of the Bankruptcy Code provides certain exemptions to allow the debtor to keep assets that are required for the debtor's basic needs. Particularly, section 522(b)(3)(C) provides that certain "retirement funds" are exempt from the bankruptcy estate – meaning they will not be used to satisfy creditors' claims. Because the Bankruptcy Code does not define "retirement funds," the Supreme Court used the ordinary meaning of the phrase, which it defined as "sums of money set aside for the day an individual stops working."

The Supreme Court considered three legal criteria of inherited IRAs to determine whether they meet the definition of "retirement funds." First, the beneficiary of an inherited IRA cannot invest additional money in the account. Second, the beneficiary of an inherited IRA must withdraw money from the account regardless of proximity to retirement. The beneficiary must either withdraw all of the funds within five years after the owner's date of death or take minimum annual distributions each year. Third, the holder of an inherited IRA may withdraw the entire balance of the account at any time without penalty. Because inherited IRAs have these features, the Supreme Court agreed with the Seventh Circuit that inherited IRAs constitute "a pot of money that can be freely used for current consumption, not funds objectively set aside for one's retirement." The Supreme Court reasoned that to allow the exemption for inherited IRAs would give the debtor a windfall, which is not the purpose of the Bankruptcy Code's exemption provisions.

On the other hand, the Supreme Court affirmed that traditional and Roth IRAs fall within the definition of exempt "retirement funds" because, unlike inherited IRAs, the owner is encouraged with tax incentives to invest funds over his or her lifetime in order to save for retirement and is required to wait until age Fifty Nine and One-Half (59 ½) before he or she can withdraw the funds without a penalty. The Supreme Court reasoned that traditional and Roth IRAs are structured to ensure that the owner will have funds to meet his or her basic needs during retirement – which is consistent with the purpose of the Bankruptcy Code's exemptions.

However, although the Supreme Court held that inherited IRAs are not protected from creditors in bankruptcy under the federal exemptions, the Bankruptcy Code allows states to opt out of the federal exemptions in favor of state exemptions. Florida is one such state that has opted out of the federal bankruptcy exemptions in favor of its own state exemptions. In particular, section 222.21(2)(a)(1), Florida Statutes, exempts traditional and Roth IRAs from claims of creditors. In 2011, the Florida legislature amended section 222.21(2)(c) to explicitly include inherited IRAs in the exemption from claims of creditors.

Therefore, although the federal bankruptcy provisions do not exempt inherited IRAs from claims of creditors, the Florida Statutes have been broadened by the legislature to include inherited IRAs. Accordingly, if the beneficiary of an inherited IRA is a Florida resident and files for bankruptcy in Florida, then the inherited IRA should be exempted from the claims of creditors under section 222.21(2)(c).

It is important to note that the domicile of the beneficiary of the IRA owner is irrelevant to whether the inherited IRA will receive creditor protection under the Florida Statutes. It is the beneficiary of the inherited IRA who must be a Florida resident at the time of petitioning for bankruptcy in Florida. However, because our society has become highly mobile, it may be difficult to predict where a beneficiary might reside at the time of the IRA owner's death. Therefore, reliance on section 222.21(2)(c), Florida Statutes, may be a poor strategy for the protection of an inherited IRA from the creditors of a beneficiary.

Trust As Beneficiary

The beneficiary of a trust may qualify as a designated beneficiary of an IRA if several conditions are met. The trust must be valid under state law. The trust must be irrevocable at the IRA holder's death. The trust must have identifiable humans as beneficiaries. The IRA custodian must receive the trust document and any other supporting document no later than October 31, in the year following the IRA holder's death. If the trust names more than one beneficiary, the beneficiary with the shortest life expectancy will be considered the designated beneficiary for determining the required minimum distribution.

Although generally an individual should be designated as the beneficiary of an IRA, the concern to protect IRA assets from the creditors of a beneficiary may provide sufficient justification to use an IRA "see-through" trust. An IRA see through trust has several advantages that arguably make its implementation a better strategy for the protection of an inherited IRA from creditors, as opposed to merely relying on the protection afforded in the Florida Statutes. One advantage of an IRA see-through trust is that it may be drafted such that the trustee is only required to distribute the required minimum distribution to the beneficiary, providing a stream of income to the beneficiary while protecting the remaining principle and accrued income. Additionally, the trustee may be given discretion as to making additional distributions of income and principle. This discretion may be limited by an ascertainable standard, such as the health, education, maintenance, and support of the beneficiary. A third advantage is that spendthrift provisions may also be written into the trust to protect the principle of the trust assets from creditors.

Under federal law, only an individual may be named as the beneficiary of an IRA. However, the Treasury Regulations permit a beneficiary of a trust will be treated as the designated beneficiary of an IRA if the trust is considered "see-though." In order for a trust to be considered see-through to the trust beneficiary, the following four (4) criteria must be satisfied: (1) the trust must be valid under state law; (2) the trust must be irrevocable or become irrevocable upon the death of the grantor; (3) the beneficiaries of the trust (who will benefit from the trusts interest in the IRA) must be identifiable in the trust instrument; and, (4) relevant documentation must be timely provided to the IRA administrator.

In addition, the see-though trust may either be drafted as a "conduit trust" or an "accumulation trust." A "trusteed IRA" is an additional form of IRA ownership that should be considered in contrast to drafting a separate conduit or accumulation trust.

Under a conduit trust, the trust terms require the trustee to pay all distributions from the IRA directly to the beneficiary. The remaindermen are not counted as beneficiaries because they are merely the successors in interest to the lifetime beneficiary. If the spouse is the sole beneficiary of the trust, the required minimum distribution may be deferred until age

70½.

Under an accumulation trust, the trust terms do not require the trustee to pay all distributions from the IRA directly to the beneficiary. For example, if the trust terms only require the trustee to pay distributions of income from the IRA to the beneficiary, then the trustee may accumulate distributions of principle from the IRA. Consequently, the remaindermen are counted as beneficiaries because they have a right to the principle of the trust and are more than mere successors in interest to the lifetime beneficiary. Unless separate shares are created for each beneficiary, the beneficiary with the shortest life expectancy is used to determine the required minimum distribution. Even if a spouse is the lifetime beneficiary of the trust, the required minimum distribution must start in the calendar year after the IRA owner's death because the spouse is not the sole beneficiary. Provide for separate IRAs for separate beneficiaries.

A trusteed IRA is a form of IRA ownership, in contrast with the more common custodial IRA. The advantage of a trusteed IRA is that it allows the IRA owner to customize the manner in which distributions are made to beneficiaries without the necessity of a separate trust. However, the ability to customize a trusteed IRA may depend on the sophistication of the bank or trust company that is providing trust services.

In the final analysis, perhaps the broader result of the Court's decision in <u>Clark</u> is to change the discussion regarding the protection of IRA assets. Although traditional and Roth IRAs will continue to receive protection under federal law from the owner's creditors, there must be a more in depth analysis of how to protect inherited IRAs from the beneficiary's creditors. Although the Florida Statutes protect inherited IRAs from creditors of Florida residents, employing an IRA see-through trust may be a more effective strategy for asset protection when there is little certainty about where beneficiaries will reside at the time the traditional or Roth IRA is converted to an inherited IRA. Accordingly, IRA owners who have concerns about the creditors of their beneficiaries should consult with an estate planning attorney regarding the creation of an IRA see-though trust.

Roth IRA

The Taxpayer Relief Act of 1997 created a new form of individual retirement plan called the Roth IRA. The earnings on a Roth IRA contribution accumulate income tax free, and qualified distributions from that IRA will be income tax free. The contributions to the Roth IRA, however, are not tax deductible.

A distribution from a Roth IRA is not subject to an income tax if this distribution does not occur until the participant reaches age 59 1/2 and it has been five years since a contribution was made to the Roth IRA. A distribution from a Roth IRA is also income tax free if made to a participant who becomes totally disabled or who withdraws up to $10,000 to buy a first home. Also, there is no income tax on a Roth IRA distribution to a beneficiary after a participant's death, even if the beneficiary is the taxpayer's estate.

Whereas the laws prior to 1998 prohibited a taxpayer from contributing to an IRA after 70 1/2 years of age, there is no age limitation on contributions to a Roth IRA, nor is there a requirement that amounts in the Roth IRA be distributed over the life of the taxpayer.

A traditional IRA can be converted to a Roth IRA. Subsequent distributions from a Roth IRA are not included in income if the contribution to which the distribution relates is a qualified distribution. A qualified distribution is one that is not made within the five tax year period beginning with the first tax year in which the individual made a contribution to the Roth IRA, and which is made on or after the date the individual became age 59 1/2 or after the death of the individual, or on account of the individual being disabled, or for a qualified special purpose distribution such as the first time home buyer expense. Distributions that do not meet the requirements for qualified distributions are included in income to the extent of earnings on contributions. Distributions made from a Roth IRA are treated as made from contributions first.

A Roth IRA permits a person to make non-deductible annual contributions of earned income up to the same limits allowed for a traditional IRA, regardless of a person's age. There is no tax on the income withdrawn from a Roth IRA if the contribution is held in a Roth IRA for at least 5 years and the taxpayer is at least 59 1/2 when the withdrawal occurs. With a few exceptions, there is an additional 10% penalty on the income withdrawn from a Roth IRA before age 59 1/2. In addition, there are no mandatory withdrawals required beginning at age 70 1/2. When a traditional IRA is converted to a Roth IRA, the amount converted (except for non-deductible IRA contribution amounts) is subject to tax in the year of the conversion. Thereafter, there will be no taxation on future income if the five year holding period for a Roth IRA is satisfied. Also, there will be no requirement that distributions begin at age 70 1/2.

IRA Contribution Limit

A taxpayer who is not a participant in a pension plan and who is under age 70 ½ can annually deduct the lesser of 100% of his or her earned income or $5,500 that is contributed to a traditional IRA. A taxpayer, who is 50 years of age or older by the end of the calendar year, can also deduct an additional $1,000 of his or her earned income contributed to a traditional IRA. This permits an older person to catch up for earlier years when he or she could not make a retirement contribution. Earned income means wages or other compensation for personal services. Gains from the sale of property, rental income, interest or dividends or

Social Security payments are not considered earned income. However, a contribution to an IRA can still be made for a spouse who does not have earned income if a joint income tax return is filed.

The rules for deducting contributions to a traditional IRA change if the taxpayer is a member of a pension plan. A single person actively participating in a retirement plan may still make a completely deductible contribution to a traditional IRA if his or her adjusted gross income does not exceed $61,000. This single taxpayer may partially deduct contributions to a traditional IRA if his or her modified adjusted gross income is between $62,000 and $71,000. This single taxpayer may not deduct any contribution to a traditional IRA if his or her modified adjusted gross income exceeds $71,000. A married taxpayer who is an active participant in a retirement plan or whose spouse is an active participant in a pension plan may still make a completely deductible contribution to a traditional IRA if the married couple's modified adjusted gross income does not exceed $95,000. Married taxpayers may partially deduct contributions to a traditional IRA if their modified adjusted gross income is between $98,000 and $118,000. Married taxpayers who are both participants in a pension plan may not deduct any contribution to a traditional IRA if their modified adjusted gross income exceeds $118,000. A married taxpayer who is not an active participant in a retirement plan and whose spouse is an active participant in a pension plan may still make a completely deductible contribution to a traditional IRA if the married couple's modified adjusted gross income does not exceed $183,000. There is a phase-out of the deduction between $183,000 and $191,000. If you file separately and did not live with your spouse at any time during the year and you have a workplace retirement plan, your IRA deduction is determined under the "single" filing status and the phase-out adjustment remains a $0 to $10,000.

The contributions to a traditional IRA and the earnings must be paid out in at least minimum required distributions according to the IRS rules, no later than April 1st after the taxpayer attains age 70 1/2. There will be an income tax on these annual distributions. With a few exceptions, there is an additional 10% penalty on the withdrawal from a traditional IRA before age 59 1/2.

By contrast, a Roth IRA can be established without any reduction by a single person who does not have annual modified adjusted gross income exceeding $116,000. This single taxpayer may partially deduct contributions to a Roth IRA, if his or her modified adjusted gross income is between $116,000 and $131,000. Married taxpayers may deduct contributions to a Roth IRA if their modified adjusted gross income is less than $183,000. Married taxpayers earning between $183,000 and $193,000 can take a partial deduction to a Roth IRA.

A Roth IRA permits a person to make non-deductible annual contributions of earned income up to the same limits allowed for a traditional IRA regardless of a person's age. There is no tax on the income withdrawn from a Roth IRA if the contribution is held in a Roth IRA for at least 5 years and the taxpayer is at least 59 ½ when the withdrawal occurs. With a few exceptions, there is an additional 10% penalty on the income withdrawn from a Roth IRA before age 59 1/2. In addition, there are no mandatory withdrawals required beginning at age 70 1/2. When a traditional IRA is converted to a Roth IRA, the amount converted (except for non-deductible IRA contribution amounts) is subject to tax in the year of the conversion.

A participant in a pension plan who earns more than the income limit for establishing a traditional IRA or a Roth IRA can still contribute earned income to a nondeductible IRA up to an amount that would otherwise be deductible. Until 2010, there was little income tax benefit to contribute to a nondeductible IRA, since the income earned was subject to taxation when withdrawn. In addition, withdrawals have to begin at age 70 1/2. However, the Tax Increase Prevention and Reconciliation Act of 2005 (TIPRA) states that for tax years beginning after December 31, 2009, the income cap that prohibited a person earning more than $100,000 from converting a traditional IRA to a Roth IRA was removed. There will be no taxation on future income if the five year holding period for a Roth IRA is satisfied. Also, there will be no requirement that distributions begin at age 70 1/2.

Estate Taxation of IRA

It is important to understand that if an employee ceased employment after 1984, the account balance in a deceased person's IRA or pension plan is subject to a federal estate tax in addition to the income tax. The pension plan benefits will not be included in the gross estate for federal estate tax purposes if the participant of a plan retired before 1983, and did not change his or her beneficiary designation form. In addition, a 5 or 10 year averaging must not be elected and the plan benefit must not be payable to the estate. If a person retired after 1982 and before 1985, and has not changed his or her beneficiary designation form, $100,000 can be excluded from his or her gross estate for federal estate tax purposes, provided that 5 or 10 years averaging was not elected and the benefits are not payable to the estate of the participant.

This federal estate tax can be deferred through the use of the marital deduction if the beneficiary of the IRA is the surviving spouse. This is accomplished through the use of the tax-deferred rollover. If there is no surviving spouse, a designated beneficiary will incur an income tax when he or she withdraws from the IRA to pay the estate tax attributable to the IRA, unless another asset can be used to pay the estate tax.

CHAPTER 4

ANNUITIES

- Definitions
- Death of Owner
- Death of the Annuitant
- Types of Annuities
- Immediate Annuities
- Life Income Annuity
- Life with Period Certain
- Deferred Annuities
- Free Look Period
- Penalty for Early Withdrawal
- Income Taxation of Annuities
- Distribution at Death
- Inappropriate Sale Practices
- Estate Taxation of Annuities

An annuity is an agreement whereby a person receives a lump sum in exchange for a promise to disburse monthly, quarterly or annual payments during the term of the agreement. These payments include a return of a portion of the premium initially deposited with the insurance company issuing the annuity, together with interest earned on the amount deposited. The person designated to receive these payments is known as the annuitant.

Definitions

There are frequently used terms and provisions when reviewing annuities. The owner is the person or entity that is entitled to the annuity. While the annuitant is alive, the owner of the annuity normally has the right before the annuity matures to change the ownership of the policy, assign the annuity, change the beneficiaries, terminate the annuity or make partial withdrawals.

When the annuity reaches the maturity date, which is also known as the annuitization date, periodic annuity payments begin. These payments are paid to the annuitant. The annuitant is the person to which all of the annuity calculations are based. Once the periodic annuity payments begin, they may not be changed nor canceled. Because the owner loses many of his options as of the annuitization date, it is essential that the annuity date be definitely stated. If this date is not noted on the declaration page of the annuity, this date should be confirmed with the insurance company.

Very often, the owner of a deferred annuity and the annuitant under it are not the same person. There may be several reasons for naming someone who is not the owner as the annuitant. The most frequent reason is that the owner who has sufficient funds to purchase an annuity is older than the maximum age allowed to qualify for the annuity. In order to purchase the annuity, the owner names a younger family member who qualifies age-wise as the annuitant.

Death of Owner

If the owner and the annuitant are the same person and the owner/annuitant dies, the annuity proceeds are distributed to the beneficiaries listed in the annuity application. If the owner and the annuitant are different people and the owner is the first to die during the accumulation period without having designated a beneficiary, the annuity is distributed to the owner's estate and not to the annuitant. Thus, the annuity proceeds are subject to probate administration and distributed in accordance with the owner's will. This may frustrate the owner's estate plan in that he or she may have increased the amounts left to other beneficiaries named in the will to compensate for the distribution of the annuity proceeds to those listed as annuitants. This result can be corrected during the owner's lifetime if the owner provides the insurance company with an Owner's Designated Beneficiary Form listing the beneficiaries the owner desires to receive the funds if he or she dies before the annuitization date. If this is done and the owner then predeceases the annuitant, the annuity proceeds will be distributed in accordance with the beneficiaries listed in this form, rather than being distributed to the owner's estate. If the beneficiary provisions are properly completed, the annuity proceeds should avoid probate. In addition, annuity proceeds owned by a Florida resident are not subject to his or her creditor claims.

Death of the Annuitant

If the annuitant dies after the annuitization date, the undistributed annuity proceeds do not belong to the owner of the annuity. Where the owner and annuitant are different persons, the primary beneficiary should be the owner and the alternate beneficiaries the persons to whom the owner would want to distribute the annuity proceeds at the owner's death. If this is done, and the annuitant predeceases the owner, the annuity proceeds would be distributed to the owner or to his or her beneficiaries.

Types of Annuities

Immediate Annuities

An immediate annuity is a contract whereby the purchaser pays a single premium at the time the annuity is issued, and within one year of the effective date the annuitant begins receiving periodic annuity payments (usually monthly or annually). While there are several options available in receiving annuity payments from immediate annuities, the two most commonly used options are:

Life Income Annuity

The first option is for payments to be received over the life of the annuitant. Payments stop and the annuity terminates at the annuitant's death. This type of payout provides the highest monthly or annual payments to the annuitant. If the entire single premium paid into the annuity has not been paid to the annuitant at his death, any unpaid amounts are forfeited to the insurance company.

Life with Period Certain

Another method of pay out is for the life of the annuitant with payments for a certain number of years guaranteed. For example, the payments can continue for life of the annuitant with a minimum of ten years of payments guaranteed. If the annuitant should die before the end of the ten-year period, the annuitant's beneficiaries will receive the balance of the payments due for the period specified. If the annuitant lives beyond the ten-year period, payments continue for his lifetime. The monthly or annual payments to the annuitant under this option are less than for the life-only option.

There are several valid reasons why an immediate annuity is purchased. One example is where the immediate annuity is used for structured settlement of a personal injury case where a life income to the injured party is the subject of the settlement. Another example is when an immediate annuity is purchased because an individual may be concerned about outliving his or her assets and wants to assure a sufficient income to pay for nursing home expenses or other expenses for his or her life. Sometimes, an immediate annuity must be purchased for Medicaid planning in order to reduce the countable assets available for a spouse's long-term custodial care in a nursing home. The immediate annuity assures the community spouse of the right to principal and income paid over no longer than the community spouse's lifetime.

Deferred Annuities

A deferred annuity is created when the purchaser pays one or more premiums over a period of time called the accumulation period. The annuity payments the annuitant will receive will begin more than one year after date of issue of the annuity contract. The time the periodic annuity payments start (called annuitization) is generally a specific time set forth in the annuity contract, which is known as the annuity date. The owner can elect to have the annuity payments start prior to the date stated in the contract. An important benefit of a deferred annuity is that during the accumulation period, the interest and/or capital gains earned on this money are tax deferred. This tax deferred accumulation will allow for a higher total return than an investment requiring taxes to be paid annually. However, this higher total return is mitigated by the fact that income taxes must be paid on the accumulated interest and capital gains when withdrawn. Unless there is a special exception that applies, the interest is considered withdrawn first and income taxes are payable during the year withdrawn. This special exception will be explained later in this chapter.

There are two major classes of deferred annuities:

Fixed Deferred Annuity. This annuity accrues interest at a fixed rate on a tax deferred basis during the accumulation period and provides for periodic payments at the time the annuity is annuitized. This fixed rate is set by the insurance company which sells the annuity. The annuity annual fixed rate is usually subject to a minimum rate of 3% or 4% which is stated in the annuity contract. Also, if the rate fixed by the insurance company is reduced over the previous year's rate by an amount stated in the annuity contract (usually 1%), the annuity contract provisions normally give the owner the right to cancel the annuity without penalty if he or she takes action within the period of time stated in the annuity contract. The owner has 30 days from receiving notice of the reduced rate in which to receive the annuity without incurring a penalty. If the annuity is canceled, any accumulated interest will be included in the owner's gross income and is subject to federal income tax for the year received, unless there is an Internal Revenue Section 1035 exchange, which is described later in this chapter.

Variable Deferred Annuity. This form of annuity is generally invested in mutual funds and accrues interest and capital gains tax deferred based on the performance of these mutual funds. One of the major benefits of holding mutual funds in a variable annuity rather than directly investing in mutual funds is that under the variable annuity, the owner can switch investments between available mutual funds without incurring capital gains taxes at the time of the switch, as would be the case in direct investments in mutual funds. However, these capital gains are taxed as ordinary income when withdrawn from the annuity and not at the lower capital gains rate. In addition, there is no stepped up basis with regard to these capital gains at the death of the annuitant. There is a penalty-free withdrawal provision in the contract (usually 10%) that can be withdrawn annually.

Free Look Period

All commercial annuity contracts issued in Florida are required to have an unconditional refund period. This period is frequently called the Free Look Period. The Florida statutes mandate a minimal period of at least 10 days for an unconditional refund starting from the date of delivery of the annuity contract. Each annuity contract has the Free Look Period shown in the contract, and is usually on the first page of the contract. This Free Look Period may last as long as 30 days, depending on the insurance company.

If a person has kept an annuity contract beyond the unconditional cancellation period, a determination should be made as to whether to continue the annuity or to pay a penalty for cancelling the annuity. Most annuity contracts contain a decreasing penalty for cancellation, usually starting at six to seven percent and annually reducing to no penalty in the sixth or seventh year. Some annuities, mainly those sold through no load mutual fund companies, have no penalty provision. Penalties will vary from insurance company to insurance company, and the annuity contract must be consulted to determine the exact penalty. In addition to the potential penalty, all accumulated interest (and capital gains in variable annuities) above the initial investment will be taxed as ordinary income. So even though an owner is beyond the penalty period, the potential income tax consequences may be sufficiently large to discourage cancellation.

Penalty for Early Withdrawal

Withdrawals from an annuity by a person under the age of 59 1/2 are subject to a 10% penalty. This provision in the Federal Income Tax was included to discourage the use of annuities as short-term tax sheltered investments. There are several exceptions to the imposition of this 10% penalty, such as a withdrawal attributable to a person dying or becoming disabled.

Income Taxation of Annuities

All annuities have a date upon which the insurance company starts paying the annuitant a periodic payment (usually monthly) under the terms of the contract. This periodic payment is called an annuity. Special tax provisions apply to these payments. A portion of each payment is a return of the original investment and not subject to income tax while the remainder is income which is subject to income tax.

All commercial annuity contracts permit the owner to withdraw up to 10% of the annuity value annually without penalty after the first year of the contract. Subject to the exception for distributions from annuity contracts issued prior to August 13, 1982, discussed below, withdrawals from annuities are taxed on a last in-first out basis. This means that if the accumulated interest and/or capital gains are considered withdrawn first, then a portion of the original investment is added if needed to bring the amount withdrawn up to 10%. In that case, the amount of the original investment included in the 10% would be considered return of investment and not subject to ordinary income tax.

In some instances, a person may own deferred annuities purchased prior to August 13, 1982. These annuities will normally have large amounts of accumulated income, making it impractical to cancel or withdraw large amounts of accumulated interest. Prior to the Tax Equity and Fiscal Responsibility Act of 1982 (TEFRA) that became effective on August 13, 1982, withdrawals from annuity contracts were treated by the Internal Revenue Service on a first in-first out basis. This means that withdrawals were considered to be first taken from the initial investment and then from accumulated income. Thus, amounts withdrawn up to the value of the initial investment are income tax free. In the event that deferred annuities were purchased prior to August 13, 1982 and partially funded prior to that date with additional funding after that date, the initial investment funded prior to August 13, 1982 may be withdrawn tax-free.

It is also important to understand that if a person initially purchased an annuity prior to August 13, 1982 and subsequently exchanged this annuity for another annuity under the Internal Revenue Section 1035 Tax Free Exchange as described in the following paragraph, the first in-first out provisions are grandfathered into the new annuity. Thus, the amounts equal to the initial investment can be withdrawn income tax free as if the new annuity was purchased prior to August 13, 1982.

Internal Revenue Code Section 1035 permits a tax-free exchange of annuity contracts provided the annuitant is the same under both contracts. If a person holds a deferred annuity with substantial accumulated interest and/or capital gains, he or she can purchase a new annuity by rolling over the value of the old annuity into the new annuity without paying income taxes on the accumulated income/capital gains. The new annuity is funded with the full value of the old annuity and no taxes are due. However, the seller receives a full commission for the new annuity and the customer usually has a new penalty period to contend with. Unless the customer holds the new annuity until the new penalty phases out, he or she may not be better off with the new annuity.

Distribution at Death

If annuity payments have not started as of the date of the annuitant's death, the entire annuity must be distributed to the beneficiary named in the contract within 5 years of the death of the annuitant. However, the designated beneficiary may elect, if such election is made within one year of the death of the annuitant, to have the proceeds of the annuity paid in periodic payments for the life of the beneficiary or for a period not exceeding the beneficiary's life expectancy. If the beneficiary is the surviving spouse of the annuitant, he or she may continue the annuity without taking any immediate distribution.

If the annuity payments have started prior to the annuitant's death, the balance of the annuity value will be distributed to the beneficiary at least as rapidly as it was being distributed to the annuitant at date of death. The beneficiary may negotiate with the insurance company for a lump sum payment, if desired. Income taxes under a lump sum distribution are computed on the basis of the lump sum amount minus the remaining investment in the contract.

If an annuity is held under a trust agreement, the income received or accrued for any taxable year is treated as ordinary income for that year and taxed as such. There is no deferral of accrued income. If the annuity is held in a Grantor Trust for the benefit of a natural person, the above general rule does not apply. The trustee is considered as an agent for the natural person who will be taxed when the payments are received. This exception also applies to an annuity held in trust where all of the trust beneficiaries are natural persons including those who have remainder interest and reversionary interest.

Inappropriate Sale Practices

It was reported at the National Academy of Elder Law Attorneys' 2010 Symposium that examples of omissions, misrepresentations, or outright falsehoods used in annuity sales presentation are:

a) "This provides an income you can't outlive", when in fact the product restricts annuitization, making it statistically unlikely that the purchaser will live long enough to receive the promised income.

b) "There is no risk," when in fact, the underlying investment can lose significant value and the purchaser can lose money under the terms of the contract, or, if there is a guarantee against loss, this is only possible by sacrificing significant investment gain.

c) "You will always have access to your money", when in reality withdrawals will generate high surrender charges for many years.

    d)   The agent fails to inform the purchaser of his or her right to a "free look".

    e)   "You need this to avoid probate", when in reality the purchaser would not be subject to probate or could avoid probate another way.

    f)   "You'll achieve tax savings", even though in some cases the purchase will result in higher taxes than the purchaser would have incurred without the sale.

There are certain characteristics that make an annuity unsuitable for the senior investor regardless of how it was sold. They are as follows:

1. The surrender penalty period lasts longer than life expectancy.

2. The surrender charges are higher than the industry norm (>7% or 8%).

3. The contract places significant barriers on the purchaser's ability to fully annuitize at any time after purchase.

4. The purchaser will have significant portions of his or her investment assets in deferred annuities after the purchase (>40%).

5. The purchaser is in a low income tax bracket, thereby making the costs and restrictions of a deferred annuity not worth the tax deferral benefit conferred by the annuity.

6. The purchaser's fixed income barely meets current expenses now, making it unsuitable to "lock up" any additional investment income in a product that only pays out income at a later date.

7. The purchaser is ill or has a history of illness, thereby implying a need for income now and not later.

8. The purchaser has little or no investment experience.

9. The purchase is a rollover of a tax deferred retirement account that was essentially free, to a new deferred annuity that provides no greater tax benefits but at a much higher cost.

10. The purchase is a rollover of a maturing annuity to another with few, if any, additional benefits, but with a new set of surrender charges and other barriers to the purchaser's money.

Florida Statute Sec. 627.4554, was amended in 2008, and is known as the "John and Patricia Seibel Act," sets standards and recommendations regarding the sale of insurance products to senior consumers who are over age 65. The act was named for a Florida couple who were sold $600,000 worth of deferred annuities, although both were in their 80's and could not access the funds for 15 years without paying large penalties. The purpose of the statute is to hold agents to a standard and impose a duty to "appropriately address the insurance needs and financial objectives of senior consumers at the time of the transaction." The statute lists 11 items of information an agent should collect. The statute requires the agent, or insurer if no agent is involved, to "make reasonable efforts to obtain":

1. Personal information, including the age and sex of the parties and the age and number of dependents;
2. Tax status of the consumer;
3. Investment objectives of the consumer;
4. The source of funds used to purchase the annuity;
5. The applicant's annual income;
6. Intended use of the annuity;
7. The applicant's existing assets, including investment holdings;
8. The applicant's liquid net worth and liquidity needs;
9. The applicant's financial situation and needs;
10. The applicant's risk tolerance and;
11. Such other information used or considered to be relevant by the agent in making a recommendation to the consumer regarding the purchase or exchange of an annuity.

Estate Taxation of Annuities

As a general rule, the value of the annuity is included in the deceased owner's federal estate tax return. If the annuity payments had not been started at the death of the owner, the full date of death value of the annuity is included in the owner's gross estate. If the Annuitant had been receiving annuity payments before death, the remaining value of the annuity as of the date of death is included in the annuitant's gross estate. This date of death value will be provided by the insurance company upon request.

CHAPTER 5

SELLING A RESIDENCE AND HOMESTEAD EXEMPTIONS

- Capital Gain Exclusion on the Sale of a Residence

- Reverse Mortgage

- Florida Documentary Stamp Tax

- Title Insurance

- Property Tax Exemptions

Capital Gain Exclusion on the Sale of a Residence

A single taxpayer can exclude up to $250,000 of the gain received on the sale of a principal residence, provided that the taxpayer has owned and occupied the residence as a principal residence for at least two of the past five years prior to the date of sale. This exclusion increases to $500,000 for married couples who meet this requirement.

A taxpayer who cannot meet these new requirements because of a change of employment or a disability is able to exclude a portion of the taxpayer's capital gain earned on the sale of a residence.

LIFE SITUATION #6

Paul and Carol purchased a residence in New York in 1960, for $30,000. They retired to Florida on January 1, 2013 to a new residence for which they then began claiming a homestead exemption. Paul and Carol would like to sell their New York residence, which now has an appraised fair market value of $300,000. Since Paul and Carol have resided in the New York residence for two of the last five years, they can exclude the entire $270,000 capital gain realized for federal income taxation purposes if they sell their New York residence by December 31, 2015 for $300,000. This is because they resided in their New York residence in 2011 and 2012. If Paul and Carol continue to reside in Florida and do not sell the New York residence by December 31, 2015, they cannot claim they lived in the New York residence for two of the past five years. If they wait to sell the residence after the year 2015, they will have to pay income tax on a capital gain of $270,000 if they sell it for appraised value subsequent to 2015 unless they return to New York and reside in their New York residence for two years of the past five years before selling it. They will need to abandon their claim for the Florida homestead exemption in the years they subsequently reside in New York. Florida has no state income tax. However, Paul and Carol should be aware that there is a state income tax in New York. Thus, any capital gain may also be subject to taxation at both the federal and New York rates.

LIFE SITUATION #7

Sally, a widow, purchased and lived in a residence in 2012, but in 2013 entered a nursing home where she has continued to reside. Sally still requires custodial care. If Sally sells her residence in 2015, she will be able to exclude the entire capital gain on the sale of her residence if the capital gain is under $250,000. There is an exception to the two-year residency requirement if the owner is physically incapable of residing in his or her residence. The law now gives the surviving spouse a $500,000 exclusion if the sale of the residence occurs not more than two years after the year of the death of the first spouse and all of the other conditions apply. If the surviving spouse remarries before the residence is sold or exchanged, this two year exclusion will not apply.

Reverse Mortgage

A reverse mortgage is a home loan that provides cash advances to a homeowner, but does not require any certain repayment until the home is sold or the surviving homeowner dies or relocates. The funds received from a reverse mortgage can be used for any purpose a homeowner deems appropriate including the additional expense related to a homeowner's assisted living or nursing home cost. The proceeds from a reverse mortgage can also be used to pay for unexpected repairs to the home due to storm damage. The proceeds from the loan could also be used to fund long-term care insurance premiums.

A reverse mortgage is different from a traditional mortgage, or a home equity line of credit, in that a homeowner must have sufficient income and little or no debt to qualify for these types of loans. In addition, the homeowner is required to make monthly mortgage payments. By contrast, a reverse mortgage is available regardless of the homeowner's current income. In addition, the homeowner creating a reverse mortgage cannot be foreclosed or forced to vacate the home because he or she does not make a mortgage payment.

The amount a homeowner can borrow on a reverse mortgage depends on the age of the youngest borrower, the current interest rate, and the appraised value of the home or the Federal Housing Administration's mortgage limits for the homeowners county, whichever is less. Generally, the more valuable the home, the older the homeowner, and the lower the interest rate, the greater the amount that can be borrowed.

While the homeowner is not required to make payments as long as the house remains his or her principal residence, the homeowner is still required to pay the real estate taxes, assessments and property insurance. When the home is sold or is no longer used as the borrower's primary residence, the borrower must repay to the lender the cash received from the reverse mortgage, plus the accrued interest and closing costs. The remaining equity in the home, if any, belongs to the borrower. None of the borrower's other assets will be affected by a reverse mortgage loan.

Until October of 2010, the only reverse mortgage that was insured by the Federal Housing Administration was the Home Equity Conversion Mortgage. (HECM). Over 493,815 senior citizens had taken advantage of FHA's Home Equity Conversion Mortgage as of May, 2010. All of the homeowners must have been age 62 and older in order to receive a Home Equity Conversion Mortgage. By contrast, a "proprietary" reverse mortgage is lent by a private company that owns the mortgage. Loan costs can vary from one type of reverse mortgage to another.

On October 4, 2010, the U.S. Department of Housing and Urban Development (HUD) and the Federal Housing Administration (FHA) introduced a new reverse mortgage program called the HECM Saver. The HECM Saver provided an option to the existing HECM program that then became known as the HECM Standard. The trade-off was that the amount the borrower can finance under the HECM Saver was reduced between 10 to 18 percent. This reduced the risk to the FHA insurance fund by reducing the principal limit or the amount of money available to the borrower.

The Home Equity Conversion Mortgage program has been changed as of September 30, 2013. These changes are expected to help manage the risk to the Federal Housing Administration's insurance fund as well as improve the safety for reverse mortgage borrowers. The changes include the consolidation of HECM Standard and HECM Saver programs into one. The changes were initiated after homeowners selecting lump-sum payments rather than periodic payouts strained the Federal Housing Administration's Mutual Mortgage Insurance Fund (MMIF). These seniors depleted their assets quickly and could not keep pace with paying property taxes and insurance payments.

The changes are authorized by the Reverse Mortgage Stabilization Act of 2013. The changes include an increase in mortgage insurance premiums and a reduction of the principal limit factors and an imposition on restrictions on the amount of money borrowers may draw down at closing and during first 12 months following closing. The maximum amount that can be accessed after September 20, 2013, is 70 percent of the loan commitment and even that will only be allowed for "mandatory and legal obligations" such as paying off an existing mortgage. A borrower who does not access his or her entire amount of funds at closing will have a lower mortgage insurance premium. Changes also include a financial assessment for all borrowers to ensure they will have the capacity and willingness to meet all their financial obligations and terms of the reverse mortgages, and a requirement of a set-aside at closing for payment of property taxes and insurance based on the results of the financial assessment. The financial assessment and property charge requirements became effective for all loans with case numbers assigned on or after Jan. 13, 2014. Changes to initial disbursement limits, single disbursement lump sum payment option, initial mortgage insurance premiums, and the initial mortgage insurance premium calculations for refinance transactions became effective for case numbers assigned on or after September 30, 2013.

It is important to remember that if funds actually drawn from a reverse mortgage are not spent in the same month as received, these funds will be counted as available assets to the community spouse or the nursing home patient. These excess assets could disqualify the nursing home spouse's Medicaid eligibility for subsequent months if the community spouse or the nursing home spouse has too many countable assets. Medicare and Social Security benefits are not affected by monies received from the reverse mortgage.

Further information regarding reverse mortgages can be obtained from the Internet at www.aarp.org. The Department of Housing and Urban Development also provides information regarding its approved lenders without cost. Approved housing counseling agencies are available for free, or at minimal cost, to provide information, counseling, and referrals to HUD's approved lenders.

Florida Documentary Stamp Tax

A documentary stamp tax must be paid to the clerk of the circuit court in the county where a parcel of real property is located before a deed transferring the ownership of that real property can be recorded in the official records of the clerk of that court. This tax is presently $.70 for each $100 of the amount paid for the real property. Thus, the sale of a home for $70,000 will give rise to a transfer tax of $490 payable to the state of Florida.

Although the contract for purchase and sale of this real property can provide otherwise, it is customary for the contract to require the seller of the real property to pay for the documentary stamps. The seller normally pays the documentary stamp tax because the seller is expected to deliver a deed that is marketable.

It is customary for the contract for purchase and sale of real property to provide that the buyer will pay the documentary stamp tax relating to the issuance of a promissory note given to borrow the money necessary to pay a portion of the purchase price. This documentary stamp tax for the privilege to issue a promissory note is $.35 for each $100. This means that if the seller accepts a promissory note from the buyer for $50,000 of the purchase price, the documentary stamp tax that the buyer will pay to the clerk of the circuit court will be $175. Likewise, if the buyer borrows some of the purchase price from a third party such as a bank, the buyer will pay this documentary stamp tax to the clerk of the court for the promissory note he or she gives to the bank.

Since the seller or the lender will want the repayment of the promissory note to be secured by a mortgage constituting a lien on the real property, there is also an intangible tax that must be paid for the privilege of giving a mortgage. The intangible tax on a mortgage is paid to the clerk of the circuit court when the mortgage is recorded in the official records. The intangible tax is presently two mills per dollar, or $2 per $1,000, on the exact dollar amount of the new mortgage. So if the buyer gives a mortgage to secure the repayment of a $50,000 promissory note, the intangible tax will be $100.

LIFE SITUATION #8

Paul and Carol wish to sell their home for $100,000. In addition to possibly paying a real estate commission, they will also be responsible for the transfer tax for the privilege of selling the real property which will amount to $700 ($.70 x $100,000). The buyer will probably be responsible for the cost to record the deed. The buyer will also be responsible for the transfer tax for the promissory note he or she gives to the bank.

Since the seller or the lender will want the repayment of the promissory note to be secured by a mortgage constituting a lien on the real property, there is also an intangible tax that must be paid for the privilege of giving a mortgage. The intangible tax on a mortgage is paid to the clerk of the circuit court when the mortgage is recorded in the official records. The intangible tax is presently two mills per dollar, or $2 per $1,000, on the exact dollar amount of the new mortgage. So if the buyer gives a mortgage to secure the repayment of a $50,000 promissory note, the intangible tax will be $100.

Title Insurance

The seller of real property or a person offering real property to secure the repayment of a loan may also be required to pay for title insurance. The purpose of title insurance is to reimburse the buyer of the real property or the owner of a mortgage against a loss in case the owner's or mortgagor's title to the real property is later determined to be defective or invalid. A new title insurance policy is issued when the present owner sells or refinances the real property, even if that owner received a title insurance policy from the previous owner.

This is because the coverage provided in a title insurance policy extends only to the owner who is being insured at the time of that particular closing. Thus, an owner's title insurance policy cannot be assigned to the next buyer of a parcel of real property.

Property Tax Exemptions

An Amendment to Florida's Constitution was approved by its voters on January 29, 2008. One of the provisions of this Amendment increases the current $25,000 homestead exemption to $50,000. However, the additional $25,000 exemption applies to the assessed value of the homestead between $50,000 and $75,000, but does not apply to the school tax levy.

Presently, a person entitled to a homestead exemption has his or her homestead assessed at just value as of January 1 of each year. However, the change in the assessment cannot exceed the lower of 3% of the assessment for the prior year or the percent of change in the Consumer Price Index for all urban consumers, U.S. City Average. Thus, homesteads often have a just value assessment and a lower taxable value assessment. The new Constitutional Amendment provides the taxpayer with the opportunity to transfer this accumulated Save-Our-Homes benefit to a new homestead may elect to do so within one year but not more than two years after relinquishing the previous homestead. If the owner moves to a home with an equal or greater value, the owner may transfer to the new home's valuation the lesser of 100% of the current Save-Our-Homes benefit or up to $500,000 of the benefit. If the owner moves to a home with a lesser value, the owner may transfer to the new home's valuation the lesser of the percentage of the current Save-Our-Homes benefit or up to $500,000 of the benefit. If two or more people own multiple homesteads (one each) and are moving into one new homestead, they may transfer the largest of the benefits to the newly established homestead up to $500,000. If two or more persons jointly own a homestead and are moving into more than one new homestead, they must divide the value of their benefit among the new homesteads based on the number of owners.

This Constitutional Amendment also limits the amount of the increase in the assessed value for non-homestead property to 10 percent per year, and at no time may the assessed value exceed the market value. The base year for assessing the 10 percent cap is 2008, which means the protection from the assessment increases began in 2009. The assessment limitation does not apply to school tax levies. This provision will expire after 2018, at which time the voters will decide whether it should be reauthorized.

PART TWO
PLANNING FOR DISABILITY

CHAPTER 6

OVERVIEW OF HEALTH CARE ADVANCE DIRECTIVES

Decisions about health care are made daily in every health care institution in every community. An individual usually makes these decisions after his or her physicians recommend treatment and provide information about the treatment. Decisions such as these may become much more difficult, however, when an individual loses his or her decision-making capacity. At such times, caregivers and family can face conflict over what medical treatment the individual would want if he or she could express a preference.

Legal documents such as living wills and powers of attorney for health care, known as advance directives, permit an individual to express his or her treatment preferences at a time when he or she has the decision-making capacity. In this way, a person ensures that his or her wishes will be followed if he or she is subsequently incapacitated.

In response to this concern, Congress enacted the Patient Self-Determination Act. This law requires hospitals, nursing homes, home health care agencies, and hospice programs to develop policies and educational programs on advance directives for patients, staff, and the community. All providers of health care services under Medicare or Medicaid are required:

1.   to provide written information to all adult patients on advance directives that can be used by them concerning health care decisions
2.   to ask whether the patient has signed an advance directive and document the response
3.   to avoid discriminating against a person on the basis of whether the person has completed an advance directive
4.   to make sure state law concerning advance directives is followed
5.   to provide staff education on advance directives

Health care providers are responsible for maintaining written policies and procedures concerning an individual's rights to make decisions about medical care. This includes the right to accept or refuse medical or surgical treatment and the right to develop advance directives. Providers are also required to ensure

1.   that there is documentation in the individual's medical record as to whether the individual has signed an advance directive
2.   that the provision of health care is not based on whether the individual has

signed an advance directive

3. compliance with state laws respecting advance directives
4. the education of staff and the community on issues concerning advance directives. An advance directive is a written instruction recognized under state law, such as a living will, health care power of attorney, and durable power of attorney. The Florida statutes also include anatomical gifts as an advance directive.

The Florida statutes require that a patient also be given information concerning pain management and palliative care when he or she discusses with the attending or treating physician, the diagnosis, planned course of treatment, alternatives, risks, or prognosis for his or her illness. If the patient is incapacitated, the information must be given to the patient's health care surrogate or proxy, court-appointed guardian or attorney-in-fact named in a durable power of attorney. Health care providers and practitioners must comply with a request for pain management or palliative care from a patient under their care. Facilities regulated under the Florida statutes must comply with pain management or palliative care measures ordered by the patient's physician.

CHAPTER 8

HEALTH CARE SURROGATE DESIGNATION

A person is presumed to be capable of making health care decisions until determined to be incapable of making such decisions. A patient is considered incapable of making health care decisions only after the patient's attending physician gives an opinion that the patient lacks the mental ability to make health care decisions or give informed consent. The attending physician will indicate this in the patient's medical chart.

Before becoming incapacitated, a person can sign a written document that names another person as a surrogate to make his or her health care decisions. This document must be signed by the person making the designation in the presence of two adult witnesses. A person physically unable to sign this document may, in the presence of two subscribing witnesses, direct that another person sign the document for him or her. The person who is to serve as the surrogate cannot serve as a witness to the signing of the document. At least one of the witnesses must be someone other than the patient's spouse or blood relative. A document designating a health care surrogate may also designate an alternate surrogate. The alternate surrogate may assume his or her duties as surrogate if the person originally named as surrogate is unwilling or unable to perform his or her duties.

A health care surrogate has the authority to make all health care decisions for the person during a time of mental incapacity. A person may designate a separate surrogate to consent to mental health treatment in the event he or she is determined by a court to be incompetent to consent to mental health treatment and a guardian advocate is appointed.

The surrogate must make all health care decisions in accordance with the previous instructions of the person for whom he or she is serving. Health care decisions include consenting, refusing to consent, or withdrawing consent to any and all health care, including life-prolonging procedures. If there is no indication of what the principal would have chosen, the surrogate may consider the patient's best interest in deciding that proposed treatments are to be withheld or that treatments currently in effect are to be withdrawn. Health care decisions also include applying for private, public, government, or veterans' benefits to defray the cost of health care. A health care surrogate also has the right to access all medical records of the person who designated him or her that are necessary for the health surrogate to make decisions involving health care and to apply for benefits.

A surrogate's authority to make health care decisions remains in effect until there is a determination that the person who signed the health care designation has regained the capacity to make medical decisions. Upon the commencement of the surrogate's authority, the patient's spouse and adult children must be notified that such an appointment has been made and that the surrogate has the authority to make decisions for the patient.

If the surrogate is not able or not willing to make health care decisions according to the patient's wishes and no alternate health care surrogate is named, the health care facility caring for the patient may seek the appointment of a health care proxy.

CHAPTER 7

LIVING WILLS

- Living Wills
- Terminal Condition, Persistent Vegetative State and End-Stage Condition
- Definition of Life-Prolonging Procedure
- Elective Procedures
- Procedure for Exercising a Living Will
- Procedure in Absence of a Living Will
- Effect of Living Wills Made Prior to October 1, 1999
- Prohibition of Mercy Killing

Living Will

A living will should not be confused with a last will and testament that directs the distribution of real or personal property after a person's death. A living will is a witnessed written document in which a person states whether a life-prolonging procedure should be withheld or withdrawn.

Terminal Condition, Persistent Vegetative State and End-Stage Condition

Prior to October 1, 1999, the Florida statutes defined a terminal condition to mean a condition caused by injury, disease, or illness from which there is no reasonable probability of recovery and which, without treatment, can be expected to cause death. The definition of a terminal condition also included a person suffering from a persistent vegetative state characterized by a permanent and irreversible condition of unconsciousness.

The 1999 Florida legislature approved a revision to this statute that states that beginning October 1, 1999, life-prolonging procedures may also be withheld or withdrawn from a person who is suffering from an end-stage condition. An end-stage condition is an irreversible condition that is caused by injury, disease, or illness which has resulted in progressively severe and permanent deterioration, and which to a reasonable degree of medical probability, treatment of the condition would be medically ineffective.

Definition of Life-Prolonging Procedure

Life-prolonging procedure means any medical procedure, treatment, or intervention that uses mechanical or other artificial means to sustain, restore, or replace a spontaneous vital function, and when applied to a patient in a terminal condition, serves only to prolong the dying process.

Prior to October 1, 1999, the providing of hydration and sustenance or the performance of any medical procedure considered necessary for comfort or to alleviate pain was not considered a life-prolonging procedure. A terminally ill patient was required to specifically decline feeding or hydration by stating in the living will that he or she considers the insertion of these tubes to also be a life-prolonging procedure. If such a statement was not made in the living will, feeding and hydration tubes would be inserted into a terminally ill patient as part of the normal care process provided by a hospital or nursing home. Therefore, it was important that a person state in his or her living will whether feeding and hydration tubes are to be withheld.

The 1999 legislature approved a revision to this statute that states that beginning October 1, 1999, life-prolonging procedures include artificially provided sustenance and hydration. Thus, a person signing a living will after October 1, 1999, who wishes sustenance and hydration, if terminally ill, will need to make this statement in his or her living will.

Elective Procedures

A living will should also state whether the person, if in a terminal condition, wants elective procedures that are not considered life-prolonging, such as radiation, chemotherapy, and dialysis. Likewise, a living will should clarify whether a person suffering from a terminal condition should be treated for secondary medical conditions such as pneumonia.

Procedure for Exercising a Living Will

Before proceeding in accordance with the living will, it must be determined that the patient is mentally or physically incapacitated and that

1. the patient does not have a reasonable probability of recovering competency so that the right could be exercised directly by the patient,

2. the patient's physical condition is terminal, or is in a persistent vegetative

state or an end-stage condition, and

3.   any limitations or conditions expressed orally or in a written declaration have been carefully considered and satisfied.

A health care surrogate, guardian, or family member does not have to seek court approval before consenting to the withdrawal or withholding of life-prolonging procedures for a terminally ill patient who has signed a living will.

There is no requirement that a judge first appoint a health care surrogate or a guardian to act on behalf of the patient before the health care provider or facility can withhold or withdraw life-prolonging procedures according to the dying patient's living will. If a terminally ill patient has signed a living will expressing his or her desire to withhold or withdraw life-prolonging procedures, but has not named a surrogate to follow his or her wishes, the attending physician may proceed as directed by the patient's living will. If there is a dispute or disagreement concerning the attending physician's decision to withhold or withdraw life-prolonging procedures, the physician cannot proceed to withhold or withdraw life-prolonging procedures pending an expedited judicial review. If a judicial review of a disputed decision is not sought within seven days following the physician's decision to withhold or withdraw life-prolonging procedures, the attending physician may follow the instructions in the patient's living will.

LIFE SITUATION #9

A terminally ill and comatose father is on a ventilator and slowly dying. The father has a living will. However, his adult children believe it is wrong to allow the withdrawal of the ventilator, because that will cause their father to die of asphyxiation. The children can only delay the father's specific instructions in his living will for seven days, unless they obtain a court ruling overriding the father's instructions within the seven days. If they do not, the physician must proceed with the removal of the ventilator.

Procedure in Absence of a Living Will

In the absence of a properly signed living will, the decision to withhold or withdraw life-prolonging procedures from a patient may be made by a health care surrogate named by the patient unless the designation limits the surrogate's authority to consent to the withholding or withdrawal of support. A surrogate cannot assert the incompetent patient's right to forgo treatment, without demonstrating each of the following:

1.   the patient does not have a reasonable probability of recovering competency,

2.   the patient suffers from a physical condition that is terminal, or is in a persis-

tent vegetative state or an end-stage condition, and

3.   that there is clear and convincing evidence that this decision would have been the one the patient would have chosen if he or she had been competent.

If a person has not signed a living will and has not named a health care surrogate, the decision to withhold life-prolonging procedures can be made by a health care proxy. However, a proxy's decision to withhold or withdraw life-prolonging procedures must be supported by a written declaration, and if not, the proxy's decision must be supported by clear and convincing evidence that the decision would have been the one the patient would have chosen had the patient been competent. If there is no indication of what the patient would have chosen, the surrogate may consider the patient's best interest in deciding that proposed treatments are to be withheld or that treatments currently in effect are to be withdrawn. The Florida statute creates an exception for persons in a persistent vegetative state, who have no advance directive and no family or friends available or willing to serve as a proxy to make health care decisions. This statute states that in such an event, life-prolonging procedures may be withheld or withdrawn by a judicially appointed guardian who is representing the best interest of the patient. The guardian and the patient's attending physician must first consult with the medical ethics committee of the facility where the patient is located. A conclusion must then be reached that the patient's condition is permanent and there is no reasonable medical probability for recovery. It must also be confirmed that the withholding or withdrawing of life-prolonging procedures is in the best interest of the patient. If there is no medical ethics committee at the facility, the facility must have an arrangement with the medical ethics committee of another facility or with a community-based ethics committee approved by the Florida Bio-ethics Network.

The case of In re Guardianship of Schiavo, 780 So.2d 176 (Fla. 2d 2001) demonstrates the difficulties of removing life supports without a living will. Nevertheless, the appellate court upheld the right of a health care proxy to make this decision without a living will. A total understanding of the issue is found in Bush v. Schiavo, 885 So.2d 321 (Fla. 2004).

Effect of Living Wills Made Prior to October 1, 1999

The 1999 Florida legislative revision states that an advance directive made prior to October 1, 1999, shall be given effect as executed. This new statute further states that all of these revisions become effective October 1, 1999, unless otherwise expressly stated. It is accordingly very important to understand that any living will created prior to October 1, 1999, must be construed according to the law in effect when the living will was signed. Thus, a person with a living will signed prior to October 1, 1999 should consider signing a new living will, to ensure that the living will is construed to include the new rights provided by the revised living will statute.

Prohibition of Mercy Killing

A terminally ill patient's exercise of his or her legal right to request medical assistance to hasten death by the withholding or withdrawal of life-prolonging procedures does not constitute a suicide. However, a patient whose treatment does not involve the use of a life-support system does not have the right to hasten his or her death with medical assistance. It is a felony in Florida for a physician or anyone else to deliberately assist another person in the commission of suicide. This distinction is based on the argument that the removal of life-support systems sustaining a terminally ill patient allows a natural death, but any other medical assistance to hasten a terminally ill person's death would result in an artificial death. The Florida Supreme Court's ruling in McIver v. Krischer 697 So.2d 97 (Fla. Sup. Ct., 1997) confirmed this distinction. The McIver, supra, case did not involve a terminally ill patient's refusing medical treatment and being allowed to die naturally. Instead, this case involved a physician's request to help a terminally ill patient die without the withholding or with-drawal of life-prolonging procedures.

In the McIver case, the trial court found that the patient was mentally competent and that he was in obviously deteriorating health, clearly suffering and terminally ill. The physician testified that he proposed to assist the terminally ill patient in committing suicide by in-travenous means. The trial judge held that the lethal medication could be self-administered by the patient after consultation and determination by the physician that the patient was competent, imminently dying, and prepared to die. In essence, the trial judge cleared the way for the physician to assist the patient in ending his life at some point in the future, when the patient subjectively decided there was no longer any hope that the brief life remaining to him would be one of satisfactory quality.

In reversing the ruling of the trial court, the majority of the Florida Supreme Court justices held in the McIver, supra, case that there is a distinction between disconnecting a respirator, which would result in death from natural causes, and the requested unnatural death by means of a death-producing agent prescribed by a physician. The Florida Supreme Court cited as the basis for its ruling the state of Florida's legitimate interest in the preservation of life, the prevention of suicide, and the maintenance of the ethical integrity of the medical profession.

The question presented to the Florida Supreme Court in the McIver, supra, case is essentially the same question that was presented to the U.S. Supreme Court in Vacco v. Quill, 117 Sup. Ct. Rptr. 2293, (U.S. Sup. Ct., 1997) and Washington v. Glucksberg 117 Sup. Ct. Rptr. 2258 (U.S. Sup. Ct., 1997). In those cases, the U.S. Supreme Court also refused to recognize an open-ended constitutional right to commit suicide. As stated in the Vacco, supra, opinion, the value to others of a person's life is far too precious to allow the individual to claim a constitutional entitlement to complete autonomy in making a decision to end that life.

The Florida Supreme Court, in the McIver, supra, case, also cited a New York Task Force report finding that those who attempt suicide, whether terminally ill or not, often suffer from depression or other mental disorders. The court noted that research indicates that many people who request physician-assisted suicide withdraw that request, if the depression and pain are treated. It also cited the Code of Medical Ethics, which states that physician-assisted suicide is fundamentally incompatible with the physician's role as a healer.

It is interesting to note that at the end of the McIver, supra, opinion, the Florida Supreme Court stated, "We do not hold that a carefully crafted statute authorizing assisted suicide would be unconstitutional." The court went on to state that this case should not be decided on the basis of the court's own assessment of the weight of the competing moral arguments. It was stated in a concurring opinion, "[t]he public would be much better served if the legislature, with significant input from the medical community, would craft appropriate exceptions to the general prohibition of assisted suicide, which include suitable standards, definitions, and procedures ensuring that the use of assisted suicide would truly be used to assist only those individuals who suffer unbearable pain in the face of certain death."

In November of 1994, the Oregon voters approved a carefully drafted referendum by a margin of 51 to 49 percent. This voter initiative states that a resident of Oregon who is 18 or older and who suffers from an incurable or irreversible disease that will reasonably result in death within six months may make a written and witnessed request to a physician for medication for the purpose of ending his or her life in a humane and dignified manner. An initiative in 1997 to repeal this statute failed. The margin against repealing this statute was 60 to 40 percent.

The Oregon statute requires the attending physician to determine that the patient is not suffering from a psychotic or psychological disorder or depression causing an impairment of judgment. If the physician determines the patient is competent, the physician must then inform the patient of the diagnosis, the prognosis, the risks related to the medicine to be prescribed, and the alternatives, including comfort care and pain control. The patient must also meet with a consulting physician, who must examine the patient and his or her relevant medical records, confirm in writing the attending physician's diagnosis that the patient is suffering from a terminal disease, and verify that the patient is capable, is acting voluntarily, and has made an informed decision. If after a waiting period of 15 days from the first request, the terminally ill patient is competent and again requests the medication to end his or her life, the physician may write the prescription, which may be filled and given to the patient after an additional two day wait.

Some 752 patients have committed physician-assisted suicide in Oregon during the 15 years the law has been in effect.

On November 4, 2008, the Washington state voters approved Initiative 1000 by a margin of 59% to 41%. This law makes it legal for doctors to prescribe a lethal dose of medication for patients with less than six months to live. Patients must make two separate requests, orally and in writing, more than two weeks apart; must be of sound mind and not suffering from depression; and must have their request approved by two separate doctors. Doctors are not allowed to administer the lethal dose. Five hundred and twenty-five patients have committed physician-assisted suicide in Washington during the 5 years the law has been in effect.

In 2010, a sharply divided Montana Supreme Court ruled that physician assisted suicide is not banned by state law. This made Montana the third state to allow the practice after Oregon and Washington. The Court found that physician assisted suicide is not illegal under state law. Instead, it found in a 4-3 decision that physician assisted suicide was not rendered illegal under state statute or by public policy concerns. The Montana Supreme Court again failed in 2014 to clarify if this practice is legal or illegal.

In 2012, the Massachusetts voters rejected a physician assisted suicide referendum by a 51% to 49% vote.

On May 20, 2013, the Vermont Legislature enacted the Patient Choice and Control at End of Life law. This law states that a physician shall not be subject to any civil or criminal liability or professional disciplinary action if the physician prescribes to a patient with a terminal condition medication to be self-administered for the purpose of hastening the patient's death and the physician affirms this fact by documenting in the patient's medical record. The law also affirms that no person shall be subject to civil or criminal liability solely for being present when a patient with a terminal condition self-administers a lethal dose of medication or for not acting to prevent the patient from self-administering a lethal dose of medication. The patient must be 18 years of age or older, a resident of Vermont, capable of making and communicating health care decisions for him/herself, diagnosed with a terminal illness that will lead to death within six months physician's diagnosis must include a terminal illness, with six months or less to live. The diagnosis must be certified by a consulting physician, who must also certify that the patient is mentally competent to make and communicate health care decisions. If either physician determines that the patient's judgment is impaired, the patient must be referred for a psychological examination. The attending physician must inform the patient of alternatives, including palliative care, hospice and pain management options.

It must be remembered that Florida statute 782.08 states that physician assisted suicide is a second degree felony, punishable by up to 15 years in prison and a fine of up to $10,000. For a state-by-state analysis of the laws governing physician assisted suicide read http://euthanasia.procon.org/view.resource.php?resourceID=000131.

CHAPTER 9

DO-NOT-RESUSCITATE ORDER

Resuscitation may be withheld or withdrawn from a patient by an emergency medical technician or paramedic if evidence of an order not to resuscitate by the patient's physician is presented to the emergency medical technician or paramedic. To be valid, an order not to resuscitate must be written on the form adopted by a rule promulgated by the Florida Department of Health. The form must be signed by the patient's physician and by the patient or, if the patient is incapacitated, the patient's health care surrogate or proxy as provided in chapter 765, court-appointed guardian as provided in chapter 744, or attorney in fact under a durable power of attorney as provided in chapter 709. The court-appointed guardian or attorney-in-fact must have been delegated authority to make health care decisions on behalf of the patient.

A person may not be denied treatment for any emergency medical condition that will deteriorate from a failure to provide such treatment at any general hospital or at any hospital that has an emergency room.

The Department of Health has developed a standardized do-not-resuscitate order which will be recognized by emergency medical service personnel, hospitals, nursing homes, assisted living facilities, home health agency personnel, and hospice workers. In addition, the Department of Health has developed a standardized do-not-resuscitate identification system with devices that signify, when carried or worn, that the possessor is a patient for whom a physician has issued an order not to administer cardiopulmonary resuscitation.

The statutes state that any health care provider will not be subject to criminal prosecution or civil liability, and will not be considered to have engaged in negligent or unprofessional conduct for withholding or withdrawing cardiopulmonary resuscitation pursuant to a do-not-resuscitate order and rules adopted by the Department of Health.

After checking that the DNRO form or bracelet is properly signed, the emergency medical service worker must identify the patient through a driver's license or other photo identification or from a witness who is in the presence of the patient. If there is any doubt about the validity of the DNRO form or bracelet or the identity of the patient, the emergency medical service personnel must begin life saving techniques, including CPR if appropriate. A DNRO may be revoked in writing, by physical destruction of the form or by verbally canceling it. Thus, a patient can withdraw the DNRO with a simple request to begin resuscitation procedures.

It is important to remember that a living will cannot be used to prevent CPR in a pre-hospital setting. This is because a living will is not a doctor's order. Since EMS personnel are in the field and without the guidance of the patient's attending physician, they need the medical authorization provided by the DNRO to withhold life-prolonging procedures. A DNRO is evidence that a physician has determined the course of treatment for a terminally ill patient.

CHAPTER 10

ABSENCE OF ADVANCE DIRECTIVES

If the patient has not signed an advance directive such as a living will or named a health care surrogate to execute an advance directive, the patient's health care decisions may be made for him or her by any of the following individuals, in the following order of priority:

1. the person appointed by a judge as the patient's guardian and who has the authority to agree to the medical treatment

2. the patient's spouse

3. an adult child of the patient or, if the patient has more than one adult child, a majority of the adult children reasonably available for consultation

4. a parent of the patient

5. an adult sibling of the patient or, if the patient has more than one adult sibling, a majority of the adult siblings reasonably available for consultation

6. an adult relative who has exhibited special care and concern for the patient and who has maintained regular contact with the patient and who is familiar with the patient's activities, health, and religious or moral beliefs

7. a close friend of the patient

A health care decision for an incapacitated patient may be made by the proxy after he or she is fully informed of the patient's medical condition. The proxy must reasonably believe the patient would have made the same health care decision under the circumstances. If there is no indication of what the patient would have chosen, the proxy may consider the patient's best interest in deciding that proposed treatments are to be withheld or that treatments currently in effect are to be withdrawn.

If a person has not signed a living will and has not named a health care surrogate, the decision to withhold life-prolonging procedures can be made by a health care proxy. However, a proxy's decision to withhold or withdraw life-prolonging procedures must be a written declaration or the decision must be supported by clear and convincing evidence that the decision would have been the one the patient would have chosen, had the patient been competent. The Florida statutes create an exception for persons in a persistent vegetative state, who have no advance directive and no family or friends available or willing to serve as a proxy to make health care decisions. The statute states that in such event, life-prolonging procedures may be withheld or withdrawn by a judicially appointed guardian with authority to consent to medical treatment. The guardian and the patient's attending physician must first consult with the medical ethics committee of the facility where the patient is located. A conclusion must then be reached that the patient's condition is permanent and there is no reasonable medical probability for recovery. It must also be confirmed that the withholding or withdrawing of life-prolonging procedures is in the best interest of the patient. If there is no medical ethics committee at the facility, the facility must have an arrangement with the medical ethics committee of another facility or with a community-based ethics committee approved by the Florida Bio-ethics Network.

CHAPTER 11

DURABLE POWER OF ATTORNEY

A durable power of attorney is a written document by which a person designates another to transact his or her business. The person intending to create the document is referred to as the principal. The person granted the authority to transact business for the principal is referred to as the attorney-in-fact or the agent. The attorney-in-fact has the full authority to perform, without prior court approval, every action authorized and specifically enumerated in the durable power of attorney. This authorization may even include the authority to sell or mortgage the principal's real property, including his or her homestead.

A durable power of attorney must be in writing and must be signed by the person intending to create it in the presence of two adult witnesses and a notary public. An existing power of attorney cannot be amended. This means that if a decision is made to change the Durable Power of Attorney the existing power of attorney will need to be revoked and a new power of attorney that contains the required amendment will have to be signed before two adult witnesses and a notary public. Before a power of attorney can be revoked, this intention must be stated by the principal in the revocation language of the new power of attorney or in another writing signed by the principal. However, the document revoking a power of attorney does not have to be witnessed or notarized unless it is going to be recorded where the person creating the revocation owns real property.

The attorney-in-fact named in a durable power of attorney may continue to transact business for the principal until the principal dies, revokes the power, or is determined by a court to be incapacitated. Incapacity is defined under this statute as the "inability of an individual to take those actions necessary to obtain, administer, and dispose of real and personal property, tangible property, business property, benefits, and income." A power of attorney is durable if it contains these words, "this durable power of attorney is not terminated by subsequent incapacity of the principal except as provided in chapter 709, Florida Statutes." It is not required that these exact words be used in the durable power of attorney.

If a court proceeding is subsequently initiated to determine the principal's incapacity, the authority granted to the agent under the durable power of attorney is suspended until this petition to determine incapacity is dismissed by the court. If the principal is determined to be incapacitated, a guardian of the property will be appointed to manage the principal's assets. However, a court may determine that certain authority granted by the durable power of attorney is to continue to be exercised by the agent.

A new Durable Power of Attorney statute became effective on October 1, 2011. Nevertheless, the provisions of the new statute state that a valid durable power of attorney signed before October 1, 2011, when the person signing the document was an adult in the presence of two subscribing witnesses and a notary public, will remain valid and enforceable as long as the provisions are not invalid under the new law. However, these signing requirements do not apply to military powers of attorneys which is valid if executed in accordance with the requirements for a military power of attorney pursuant to 10 United States Code section 1044(b).

The new statute states that a "springing" durable power of attorney can not be established after October 1, 2011. However, any springing durable power of attorney signed prior to October 1, 2011, will remain valid after October 1, 2011. The springing durable power of attorney was a document conditioned upon the person creating this durable power of attorney lacking the capacity to manage property as defined in the Florida guardianship statute. This definition means that a person lacks the capacity to take those actions necessary to obtain, administer, and dispose of real and personal property, intangible property, business property, benefits and income. While a judicial determination that this person lacks the capacity to manage property was not required, the statute stated that this springing durable power of attorney can only be exercised by the agent upon the delivery of the primary physician's affidavit to the third party intending to transact business with the agent, such as a bank. This affidavit had to state that this physician is licensed to practice medicine in the state of Florida, that he or she is the primary physician who has the responsibility for the treatment and care of the person who created the durable power of attorney, and that the person creating the durable power of attorney lacks the capacity to manage property as defined in the applicable Florida guardianship statute.

Florida's new Durable Power of Attorney statute states that powers of attorneys signed under the laws of another state will be valid in Florida if they are signed pursuant to the law of that state. However, a bank has the right to request its attorney to give an opinion regarding the out-of-state power of attorney being valid. The bank has the right to charge the principal or agent for this legal opinion. Nevertheless, a durable power of attorney signed in another state must be signed before two witnesses and have a notary's acknowledgment in order to convey or mortgage homestead real property.

The agent named in a durable power of attorney must be a natural person who is 18 years of age or older or a financial institution. The financial institution must have a place of business in Florida and be authorized by statute to conduct trust business in this state. The agent must agree to serve under the power of attorney by signing an acceptance if that is the method set forth in the document. If no method for agreeing to serve is described, an agent may accept his duties by performing actions authorized in the document.

A durable power of attorney may state that one person may serve as the agent or two or more persons may serve as co-agents. Each co-agent may act independently of the other agent or agents, unless the document states otherwise. If a person declines to serve as the agent or dies or resigns, one or more successor agents named in the document may then serve. It is important to understand that the authority to designate a successor agent is limited to the principal. This authority may not be delegated by the principal to anyone else. The agent's authority is also terminated upon the filing of an action for dissolution, legal separation, or annulment of the marriage of the agent to the principal or if the principal is adjudicated totally or partially incapacitated.

An agent named in a durable power of attorney is entitled to be reimbursed by the principal for his or her reasonable costs and expenses. Only a qualified agent or a natural person who is a resident of Florida, and not in the business of serving as an agent can be paid for his or her services. The new Florida statute defines a qualified agent as a financial institution with trust powers that has a place of business in Florida, an attorney or certified public accountant licensed in Florida, the principal's spouse, and any heir of the principal. Relatives of the last deceased spouse of the principal qualify as heirs of the principal. A qualified agent can also be any other natural person, provided the person is a resident of Florida and the person is not in the business of serving as an agent. A person who has been an agent for more than three principals at the same time is considered to have been in the business of serving as an agent and cannot receive compensation.

The new Florida statute governing durable powers of attorney states that beginning October 1, 2011, certain authorities must be specifically granted. These powers are referred to as the "superpowers." A common thread to these superpowers is that their exercise can impact a principal's existing estate plan. These rules do not affect pre-Act powers of attorney signed prior to October 1, 2011. If specifically authorized, the agent may on the principal's behalf exercise these superpowers:

- Create an inter vivos trust;
- Amend, modify, revoke or terminate a trust created by or on behalf of the principal;
- Make a gift;
- Create or change rights of survivorship;
- Create or change a beneficiary designation;
- Waive the principal's right to be a beneficiary of a joint and survivor annuity, including a survivor benefit under a retirement plan; or
- Disclaim property and powers of appointment.

To ensure that the principal knows he or she is granting these special powers to the agent, the new statute requires that the principal place his or her signature or initials next to the paragraph containing the enumeration of the agent's authority of a power. It is not enough for the principal to sign or initial the page on which these powers appear. Because a gift of the principal's property reduces the principal's estate, the Act sets a default per-donee limit on gift amounts. Unless the authorization provides otherwise, gifts by the agent may not exceed the annual exclusion amount that is presently $14,000 per person (or twice that amount in the case of a split gift).

The new statute states that third persons may require an agent to execute an affidavit as to the agent's knowledge regarding the effectiveness of the power of attorney and the agent's authority. The section specifically provides that the following facts are appropriate for the affidavit, although this list should not be deemed exclusive:

- The domicile of the principal;
- That the principal is not deceased;
- That there has been no revocation, or partial or complete termination of the power of attorney, either by adjudication of incapacity or some other event identified in the instrument;
- That there has been no suspension of the power of attorney by the filing of proceedings to determine the principal's capacity or to appoint a guardian or guardian advocate;
- How the agent succeeded to the position if the agent is a successor.

CHAPTER 12

PLANNING FOR PETS

A person's estate and disability plan can include directions regarding the disposition of his or her pets in the event that the owner dies or becomes disabled. The pet owner's durable power of attorney can provide that during the owner's extended illness or incapacity, the agent named in the durable power of attorney is authorized to pay the bills required for the care of the owner's pets. The durable power of attorney can specify the type of care authorized for the pets. The durable power of attorney can include authorization for paying for the pets' regular exercise, grooming, veterinary care and special dietary needs, if any.

A person's disability planning documents can also state that it is his or her intention for the household pets to remain in the home with the owner as long as it is medically advisable. If a revocable trust has been established, a successor trustee can be directed in this instrument to pay for the pets' regular exercise and medical care if the owner can no longer provide this care. The successor trustee can also be authorized to pay family members or friends for the time they expend in attending to the pets. In the alternative, a successor trustee can be specifically authorized to employ pet care professionals to arrange for the pets' regular exercise and companionship. For instance, the trust can state that professional pet sitters can come to the home to exercise a dog and attend to a cat or another pet. The trust can also state which veterinary clinic has attended to these animals and direct that this veterinary clinic should continue to care for these animals if the owner becomes incapacitated.

A person's disability planning documents can state that in the event that a person is forced to leave home because of his or her medical condition, the health care surrogate may select an adult family care home or other assisted living facility for the owner which permits his or her pets to stay with the owner. If that is not possible, the health care surrogate can be instructed to arrange for the owner's regular visits with his or her pets. It is, of course, important to state that this is the owner's intention with regard to household pets such as small house size dogs, cats or birds. This will prevent unusual pets or barnyard animals from being included in this care plan.

A separate concern arises regarding what will become of an owner's pets after his or her death. A person's last will and testament can direct who will take an owner's pets after his or her death. A will or revocable trust can direct that the person named to take the pets be given sufficient funds to support the pets during their natural lifetime. However, there is no guarantee that this care provider will actually use the funds to support a deceased person's pets, unless a trust fund is established for this purpose.

The will or trust provisions regarding the pet could state that if the person being left the pet and the right to receive money to care for the pet's medical care and support is unable or unwilling to care for the pet, this gift will lapse. In such event, the personal representative (executor) or trustee should be directed to arrange for a suitable home for the domestic pet and to prepay the projected medical care and food costs for the projected lifetime of the pet.

Another solution might be to prepay the pet's medical care pursuant to a contract with a veterinarian and to establish a lifetime care contract arrangement with a veterinarian or dog care manager (similar to a geriatric care manager) to oversee the pet's new home situation. It may also be possible to contract with a charitable organization that will agree to feed and shelter a survivor's pet in exchange for a cash contribution.

The Florida legislature has approved legislation permitting a person to establish a trust for the care of a deceased person's animals. The new legislation states that a trust may be created to provide for the care of an animal alive during a person's lifetime. The trust terminates upon the death of the animal, or if the trust is created to provide for the care of more than one animal alive during the person's lifetime, upon the death of the last surviving animal. Unless a trust document provides otherwise, the Florida statutes regarding the administration of a trust will apply to a trust for the care of an animal.

The property of a trust authorized by this law may be applied only to its intended use for the animals. However, the law states that a circuit judge may determine whether the value of the trust property exceeds the amount required for the projected expense for the animals. The law states that trust property determined by the circuit judge cannot be required for this intended use, and any trust property remaining upon the trust's termination due to the animal's death shall be distributed as directed to the ultimate beneficiaries named in the trust.

CHAPTER 13

BAKER ACT

- Baker Act

- Guardian Advocate For Baker Act Proceedings

Baker Act

The purpose of Florida's mental health statute known as the Baker Act is to provide examination and short-term treatment for a person suffering from a mental illness. This statute also authorizes the court to order continued placement in certain circumstances if the person, because of his or her mental illness, suffers from self-neglect or is dangerous to self or others.

The intent of this statute is for a person in need of mental health treatment to be admitted as a patient to a facility on a voluntary basis, if competent to give express and informed consent to treatment. However, the statute also provides for involuntary placement, but only after authorized mental health professionals and a circuit judge confirm it is necessary. The primary goal of the statute is to ensure that individual dignity and human rights are guaranteed to any person admitted as a patient to a mental health facility.

An involuntary psychiatric examination may be initiated by a law enforcement officer who has reason to believe a person appears to meet the criteria for an involuntary examination. It may also be initiated by an order of a circuit judge, if the application filed by one or more persons with the clerk of the court provides sufficient reason to believe another person is in need of a psychiatric examination. In addition, a request for an involuntary psychiatric examination can be initiated by a physician, clinical psychologist, psychiatric nurse, or licensed clinical social worker who has observed that person within the preceding 48 hours and finds (as a result of the observation) that the person meets the criteria for an involuntary examination.

The basis for the involuntary examination is if the person to be examined is mentally ill and without care or treatment, the person is likely to suffer from neglect or refuse to care for his or her self, or is likely to cause bodily harm to his or her self or others. This neglect or refusal of care must pose a real and present threat of substantial harm to the person's well-being. The mentally ill person must be refusing voluntary examination or be unable to determine whether examination is necessary. It must also be apparent that harm to the person cannot be avoided through the help of willing family members or friends.

If the judge issues what is called an ex-parte order or if the professional signs a certificate stating that a person needs to be examined, the law enforcement officer must deliver the person to the nearest facility designated to receive patients under emergency conditions for a psychiatric evaluation. The person is then examined without unnecessary delay by a physician or clinical psychologist and may be given emergency treatment for the safety of the person or others. The person may not be detained at the facility for more than 72 hours. Within the examination period, the patient must be released or may give expressed and informed consent to continued voluntary placement, or a petition for involuntary placement must be signed by the facility administrator and filed with the clerk of the court. If a petition for involuntary placement is filed, a circuit judge or a hearing master appointed by the circuit judge must hold a hearing within five days to determine whether there is clear and convincing evidence to believe that the patient meets the criteria for involuntary placement. The maximum period for an involuntary commitment is six months.

At any time, a person held in a mental health facility or a relative, friend, guardian, guardian advocate, representative or attorney, or the Department of Children and Families, on behalf of such person may petition for a writ of habeas corpus to question the cause and legality of such detention. The petitioner can allege that the patient is being unjustly denied a right or privilege granted by law. The petitioner can request that the circuit court issue an order directing the hospital to respond to the writ.

Significant mental health laws relate to the voluntary admission to a mental health facility of a person 60 years of age or older who is presently residing at a nursing home, assisted living facility, adult day care center or adult family care home and has previously been diagnosed as suffering from dementia. The statutes provide that an initial assessment of the patient's ability to give informed consent to treatment is necessary before the person can be transferred from the care facility and admitted on a voluntary basis to a mental health facility.

This initial assessment must be performed by a state designated crisis service at the facility where the patient is residing. This requirement also applies to the voluntary admission of a person to a facility from a nursing home, assisted living facility, adult day care center, or adult family care home when all decisions concerning medical treatment are currently being made by a health care surrogate or proxy. If the designated crisis service cannot respond, the assessment may be performed by an authorized licensed professional who is not employed or under contract, and does not have a financial interest in either the facility initiating the transfer nor the receiving facility to which the transfer may be made.

The statutes further state that within 24 hours after the voluntary admission of any patient to a treatment facility, the admitting physician must document in the patient's clinical record that the patient is able to give informed consent for admission. If the patient is not able to give consent, the facility must discharge the patient or transfer him or her to involuntary status. Transferring the patient to involuntary status will assure that the patient receives a court hearing regarding his or her need for continued treatment.

The statutes governing nursing homes, assisted living facilities, adult day care centers, and adult family care homes state that action may be taken by the Agency for Health Care Administration against such a facility for failure to follow the criteria and procedures provided in these mental health statutes. This action includes the right to deny, revoke, or suspend a license or to impose an administrative fine.

Guardian Advocate For Baker Act Proceedings

The Baker Act statute provides that when a mentally ill person is involuntarily committed to a facility, a person known as a guardian advocate must be appointed by the court to make decisions regarding mental health treatment on behalf of a patient, if the patient is found incompetent to consent to treatment. The Baker Act statute provides that the court should give preference in the appointment of a guardian advocate to the person designated to make health care decisions in a health care surrogate designation. If the patient has not previously designated a health care surrogate, preference is then given to the patient's spouse. If there is no spouse, then the following priority should be applied in appointing a guardian advocate:

1. an adult child of the patient
2. a parent of the patient
3. the adult next of kin of the patient
4. the adult friend of the patient
5. an adult trained and willing to serve as the guardian advocate

The Baker Act statute also states that, unless the requirement is waived by the court, a guardian advocate must, prior to exercising his or her authority, attend a training course approved by the court. The training course must be a minimum of four hours and must include information about psychotropic medications that affect a person's mental state, diagnosis of mental illness, the ethics of medical decision making, and duties of guardian advocates.

It is important to know that the Florida statutes state that a person may designate a separate surrogate to consent to mental health treatment if he or she is later determined by a court to be incompetent to consent to mental health treatment and a guardian advocate is appointed. However, unless the document designating the health care surrogate specifically states otherwise, the court assumes that the surrogate authorized to make health care decisions may also make decisions regarding mental health treatment.

CHAPTER 14

GUARDIANSHIPS

Any adult may file a petition requesting that a circuit judge determine the incapacity of another person with the clerk of the circuit court in the county where the alleged incapacitated person resides or is found. The circuit judge will then appoint an examining committee consisting of three members. One member must be a psychiatrist or other physician. The remaining members consist of a psychologist, another physician, a registered nurse, nurse practitioner, a licensed social worker or other persons who by knowledge, skill, experience, training or education advise the court in the form of an expert opinion. One of the three members of the committee must have knowledge of the type of incapacity alleged in the petition. The circuit judge must also appoint an attorney to represent the person alleged to be incapacitated.

If the examining committee decides that the person is not incapacitated in any respect, the circuit judge must dismiss the petition for incapacity. If the examining committee decides that the person is incapacitated in any respect, a hearing will be held by a circuit judge. The person assumed to be incapacitated must be present at the hearing, unless this right is waived by the alleged incapacitated person or his or her attorney, or unless good cause can be shown for the alleged incapacitated person's absence.

A person may be determined to be incapacitated by a court of law when he or she lacks the ability to manage at least some of his or her property or to attend to at least some of his or her essential health and safety requirements. A person is considered unable to manage his or her property if he or she cannot take the necessary actions to obtain, administer, and dispose of his or her real and personal property. A person is considered unable to meet the essential requirements for health or safety if he or she cannot take the necessary actions to provide health care, food, shelter, clothing, personal hygiene, or other care without which serious and immediate physical injury or illness can occur.

The alleged incapacitated person's incapacity must be established by clear and convincing evidence. After hearing all the evidence, the circuit judge may still dismiss the petition if there is insufficient evidence to support a finding of incapacity. However, a circuit judge may determine a person to be totally incapacitated if he or she is incapable of exercising all of his or her non-delegable and delegable rights. Non-delegable rights are the right to marry, vote, personally apply for government benefits, have a driver's license, travel, or seek and retain employment. Delegable rights are the right to contract, sue and defend lawsuits, apply for government benefits, determine residency, consent to medical and mental health treatment, manage property, or make gifts of property or decide social environment or other social aspects of life. The judge will then assign the incapacitated person's delegable rights to a guardian appointed by the judge.

A competent adult may designate in advance the person whom he or she wants to subsequently be his or her guardian, by signing a written document that names a person to serve as his or her guardian in the event of a subsequent incapacity. The written declaration must reasonably identify this pre-need guardian and be signed in the presence of at least two attesting witnesses.

A person may file his or her declaration with the clerk of the court. If a petition for incapacity is subsequently filed, the clerk of the court must produce this declaration to the circuit judge. The presentation of such a declaration in an incapacity proceeding establishes a rebuttable presumption that the pre-need guardian should serve as the guardian. However, the circuit judge is not bound to appoint the pre-need guardian if this named person is determined by the circuit judge to be unqualified to serve as the guardian.

When a person is appointed the guardian of an incapacitated person's property, a bond must be posted before beginning to serve as guardian for at least the full amount of the ward's cash on hand and on deposit, the value of the ward's promissory notes and bonds and the value of all other intangible personal property, such as stocks, that can readily be traded for cash. The bond must be filed with the clerk before a person can begin to serve as the guardian of the property. The amount of the bond can be lowered as the guardianship assets subsequently dissipate. Even if the ward had the right to revoke the trust, the assets previously transferred to a trust are not considered guardianship assets. The assets owned by a trustee of the ward's revocable trust are not counted in determining the amount of the guardianship assets subject to a bond.

If a petition to determine the incapacity of a person is filed, the right of the agent to use the durable power of attorney is suspended until the circuit judge determines the capacity of the person who established the durable power of attorney. If a finding is made that the person who signed the durable power of attorney is incapacitated, the durable power of attorney will remain suspended until the capacity of the person who signed this durable power of attorney is restored.

In each proceeding in which a guardian is appointed, the circuit judge must determine whether the ward, prior to incapacity, executed a valid advance directive. An advance directive is a witnessed written document in which instructions are given or in which a person's desires are expressed concerning any aspect of his or her health care. An advance directive may include, but is not limited to, the designation of a health care surrogate. If any such advance directive exists, the court shall specify in its order of guardianship what authority, if any, the guardian shall exercise over the surrogate or agent named in the advance directive. The court may, with prior notice of a hearing given to the surrogate and other interested parties, subsequently modify or revoke the authority of this surrogate or agent to make health care decisions.

CHAPTER 15

DEVELOPMENTAL DISABILITIES

A "Developmental disability" means a disorder or syndrome that is attributable to intellectual disability, cerebral palsy, autism, spina bifida, or Prader-Willi syndrome; that manifests before the age of 18; and that constitutes a substantial handicap that can reasonably be expected to continue indefinitely.

A person with a developmental disability may not be presumed incapacitated solely by reason of his or her acceptance in nonresidential services or admission to residential care and may not be denied the full exercise of all legal rights guaranteed to citizens of this state and of the United States.

A circuit court may appoint a guardian advocate, without an adjudication of incapacity, for a person with developmental disabilities, if the person lacks the decision making ability to do some, but not all, of the decision making tasks necessary to care for his or her person or property or if the person has voluntarily petitioned for the appointment of a guardian advocate.

A petition to appoint a guardian advocate for a person with a developmental disability may be signed by an adult person who is a resident of this state. The petition must be verified and must allege that the petitioner believes that the person needs a guardian advocate and specify the factual information on which such belief is based. The petition must also state the exact areas in which the person lacks the decision making ability to make informed decisions about his or her care and treatment services or to meet the essential requirements for his or her physical health or safety. The petition must also specify the legal disabilities to which the person is subject.

Notice of the filing of the petition to appoint a guardian advocate must be given to the person with a developmental disability, verbally and in writing in the language of the person and in English. Notice must also be given to the next of kin of the person with a developmental disability, a health care surrogate, an agent under a durable power of attorney. A copy of the petition to appoint a guardian advocate must be served with the notice. The notice must state that a hearing will be held to inquire into the capacity of the person with a developmental disability to exercise the rights enumerated in the petition. The notice must also state the date of the hearing on the petition.

Within 3 days after a petition has been filed, the circuit judge must appoint an attorney to represent a person with a developmental disability who is the subject of a petition to appoint a guardian advocate. The person with a developmental disability may substitute his or her own attorney for the attorney appointed by the court.

Upon the filing of the petition to appoint a guardian advocate, the court must set a date for holding a hearing on the petition. The hearing must be held as soon as practicable after the petition is filed, but reasonable delay for the purpose of investigation, discovery, or procuring counsel or witnesses may be granted.

The person with a developmental disability has the right to be present at the hearing and shall be present unless good cause to exclude the individual can be shown. The person has the right to remain silent, to present evidence, to call and cross-examine witnesses, and to have the hearing open or closed, as the person may choose. The burden of proof must be by clear and convincing evidence.

The court shall determine whether the person with a developmental disability has executed any valid advance directive or a durable power of attorney. If the person with a developmental disability has executed an advance directive or durable power of attorney, the circuit judge must consider and find whether the documents will sufficiently address the needs of the person with a developmental disability for whom the guardian advocate is sought. A guardian advocate may not be appointed if the court finds that the advance directive or durable power of attorney provides an alternative to the appointment of a guardian advocate which will sufficiently address the needs of the person with a developmental disability. If an advance directive exists, the court shall specify in its order and letters of guardian advocacy what authority, if any, the guardian advocate shall exercise over the person's health care surrogate. The court, upon its own motion, may, with notice to the health care surrogate modify or revoke the authority of the health care surrogate to make health care decisions for the person with a developmental disability. If any durable power of attorney exists, the circuit judge shall specify in its order and letters of guardian advocacy what powers of the agent, if any, are suspended and granted to the guardian advocate. The circuit judge, however, may not suspend any powers of the agent unless the judge determines the durable power of attorney is invalid or there is an abuse by the agent of the powers granted.

If the circuit judge finds the person with a developmental disability requires the appointment of a guardian advocate, the judge must enter a written order appointing the guardian advocate and containing the findings of facts and conclusions of law on which the court made its decision, including the nature and scope of the person's lack of decision making ability, the exact areas in which the individual lacks decision making ability to make informed decisions about care and treatment services or to meet the essential requirements for his or her physical health and safety, the specific legal disabilities to which the person with a developmental disability is subject, the name of the person selected as guardian advocate and the reasons for the court's selection and the powers, duties, and responsibilities of the guardian advocate, including the bonding of the guardian advocate.

The guardian advocate for a person with a developmental disability shall be a person or corporation qualified to act as guardian, with the same powers, duties, and responsibilities required of a guardian appointed under an incapacity proceeding or those defined by the court order. However, a guardian advocate may not be required to file an annual accounting if the court determines that the person with a developmental disability receives income only from Social Security benefits and the guardian advocate is the person's representative payee for the benefits.

Any interested person, including the person with a developmental disability, may subsequently file a suggestion of restoration of rights with the court in which the guardian advocacy is pending. The suggestion must state that the person with a developmental disability is currently capable of exercising some or all of the rights that were delegated to the guardian advocate and provide evidentiary support for the filing of the suggestion. Evidentiary support includes, but is not limited to, a signed statement from a medical, psychological, or psychiatric practitioner by whom the person with a developmental disability was evaluated and which supports the suggestion for the restoration. Within 3 days after the filing of the suggestion, counsel shall be appointed for the person with a developmental disability.

If no objections are filed and the court is satisfied with the evidentiary support for restoration, the court shall enter an order of restoration of rights which were delegated to a guardian advocate and which the person with a developmental disability may now exercise. At the conclusion of a hearing, the court shall enter an order denying the suggestion or restoring all or some of the rights that were delegated to the guardian advocate. If only some rights are restored to the person with a developmental disability, the court shall enter amended letters of guardian advocacy.

CHAPTER 16

ADULT FAMILY-CARE HOME

There comes a point in time when a disabled adult or a frail elder may prefer to live with an individual or family in a private home. This person does not need custodial or skilled care that is provided in a nursing home and may not wish to reside in an assisted living facility. However, this disabled adult or frail elder will need clean and sanitary accommodations and some personal services provided in an adult family-care home. This homelike environment should also promote the dignity, individuality, and privacy of the resident while retaining his or her decision-making ability.

Such a facility is defined by the Florida statutes as an adult family-care home. This full-time family-type living arrangement is provided by a person who owns or rents the home that delivers room, board, and personal care, on a 24-hour basis to no more than five disabled adults or frail elders who are not relatives. A disabled adult is defined by statute to mean any person between 18 and 59 years of age who has one or more permanent physical or mental limitations that restrict his or her ability to perform normal activities of daily living. A frail elder means a functionally impaired person who is 60 years of age or older and has physical or mental limitations that restrict his or her ability to perform the normal activities of daily living and that impede the person's capacity to live independently.

A person who intends to operate an adult family-care home which provides the housing, meals, and personal care to three or more adults must first obtain a license from Florida's Agency for Health Care Administration. This license is effective for one year and must be renewed annually. In addition, the person who provides these services must actually reside at this residence. Such a facility is not required to be licensed as an adult family-care home if the person who owns or rents the home provides room, board, and personal services for no more than two adults who do not receive supplemental housing assistance from Florida's Department of Children and Families. Another exception to the licensing requirement is when the person who owns or rents the home provides the room, board and personal services only to his or her relatives.

Florida's Agency for Health Care Administration in consultation with the Department of Health, the Department of Elder Affairs, and the Department of Children and Families is charged with establishing minimum standards to ensure the health, safety, and well-being of each resident in an adult family-care home. These rules provide that in order to be admitted to an adult family-care home, a resident must be capable of self-preservation in an emergency situation involving the immediate evacuation of the adult family-care home, with assistance in ambulation if needed. The resident must also be able to perform, with supervision or assistance, his or her activities of daily living and not be a danger to self or others. The resident must not be bedridden or require the use of chemical or physical restraints and not require 24-hour nursing supervision.

The provider of the services, all staff, each relief person and all household members of an adult family-care home must be screened for criminal histories. A background check is performed by the Florida Department of Law Enforcement to confirm that the owner, relief persons, all adult household members, and employees of the adult family-care home have not been found guilty of certain criminal offenses.

The Florida statutes provide each resident of an adult family-care home with a resident's bill of rights. This means that an adult family-care home may not deprive a resident of his or her civil or legal rights. In addition, each resident has the right to be free from abuse and neglect. Each resident is entitled to keep and use his or her own clothes.

A resident is also entitled to unrestricted private communication, including receiving and sending unopened correspondence, having access to a telephone and visiting with any person of his or her choice at any time between the hours of 9 a.m. and 9 p.m., at a minimum. The resident must receive at least 30 days notice of relocation or termination of residency from the home unless, for medical reasons, the resident is certified by a physician to require an emergency relocation to a facility providing a more skilled level of care or the resident engages in a pattern of conduct that is harmful or offensive to other residents. A resident whose rights are violated has a cause of action against the adult family-care home, provider or staff responsible for the violation.

Before or at the time of admission to an adult family-care facility, the provider and the resident must sign a residency agreement which includes a list specifically setting forth the services and accommodations to be provided, the daily, weekly and monthly rates and charges, and a statement that the provider will provide at least 30 days notice before implementing a rate increase. The agreement must set forth the discharge policy and provide for a refund policy if the resident is discharged or dies.

A resident of an adult family-care home is allowed the free use of all space within the home except when such use interferes with the safety, privacy and personal possessions of household members and other residents. Single bedrooms for residents must provide at least 80 square feet of floor space for each resident. Multi-occupancy bedrooms must provide at least 60 square feet of floor space per person. An adult family-care home must have a yard which is available and accessible by the residents.

Similarly, an elderly person or an adult with a disability may decide to reside in an assisted living facility. An assisted living facility also provides housing, meals and one or more personal services for periods exceeding 24 hours. Legislation governing assisted living facilities is intended to encourage the development of innovative and affordable facilities while ensuring that the needed economic, social mental health, health and leisure services are made available to residents of such facilities.

CHAPTER 17

NURSING HOME PATIENT RIGHTS

- Nursing Home Discharges
- Resident's Rights
- Office of the State Long-Term Care Ombudsman
- Selecting a Nursing Home

Nursing Home Discharges

The Florida statutes state that a nursing home's ability to transfer or discharge a resident for whom payment is being received is restricted to only medical reasons or for the welfare of other patients. Likewise, a Medicaid-certified or Medicare-certified nursing home can only involuntarily transfer or discharge a resident for the following reasons:

1. The transfer or discharge is necessary for the resident's welfare because the resident's needs cannot be met in the facility.
2. The transfer or discharge may be appropriate because the resident's health has improved to such a degree that the resident no longer needs the services provided by the facility.
3. The health or safety of other residents or facility employees is endangered.
4. The resident has failed to pay for the stay in the facility.
5. The facility has ceased to operate as a nursing home.

The fact that there is an additional burden to the nursing home is not a sufficient basis for discharge of a patient. If a nursing home is proposing to discharge a patient because he or she requires an extraordinary amount of care, the nursing home administrator should be asked to make a reasonable accommodation for the patient's individual needs. This may necessitate additional staffing by the nursing home or a change in the staff's routine to better address the patient's needs. An inquiry should be made to determine whether there are other residents in the nursing home who require and are receiving the same care needed by this resident.

If the nursing home staff continues to assert that a resident will be better cared for at another facility, that nursing home has a responsibility to provide proper discharge planning for the resident. This includes locating another nursing home with a vacancy for the suitable placement of the resident. In addition, the nursing home must provide sufficient preparation and orientation of the resident to ensure a safe and orderly transfer from the facility. An example might include a trial visit by the resident to the new nursing home location and a briefing of the staff at the new nursing home of the resident's daily needs.

If the nursing home insists on transferring a patient to another nursing home but the patient's caregiver or family does not believe the transfer is necessary, the caregiver or the family of a resident of any Medicaid-certified or Medicare-certified facility may challenge a decision by that facility to discharge or transfer the resident. At least 30 days prior to any proposed transfer or discharge, the facility must provide advance notice of the proposed move to the resident and to a family member, or to the resident's legal representative, if known. The nursing home statute provides that a resident is entitled to a hearing by the Department of Children and Families Office of Appeals to challenge a facility's proposed transfer or discharge. Unless the discharge or transfer constitutes an emergency, a written request by the resident for a fair hearing within 10 days from receiving the notice of the intended transfer from the facility will stay the proposed transfer pending the decision. The fair hearing must be completed within 90 days of receipt of the resident's request.

If the patient fails to timely request a hearing within 10 days of receipt of the facility's notice of the proposed move, the facility may transfer or discharge the patient after 30 days from the date he or she received the notice. If the hearing decision is favorable to the patient who has been transferred or discharged, the facility must readmit him or her to the facility's first available bed.

Florida's nursing home laws state that a nursing home's written notice of its intention to discharge a patient must state the means for a resident to request the local long-term ombudsman council to review the notice and request information about or assistance with the initiating of a fair hearing with the Department of Children and Families Office of Appeals. In addition, the form must specify the reason allowed under federal or state law that the resident is being discharged or transferred, with an explanation to support this action. Further, the form must state the effective date of the discharge or transfer and the location to which the resident is being transferred or discharged. The form must describe the resident's appeal rights and the procedures for filing an appeal, including the right to request the local ombudsman council to review the notice of discharge or transfer.

A resident may request that the local ombudsman council review any notice of discharge or transfer given to the resident. When requested by a resident to review the notice of discharge or transfer, the local ombudsman council must do so within 7 days after receipt of the request. The nursing home administrator's designee must forward the request for review contained in the notice to the local ombudsman council within 24 hours after the request is submitted. Failure to forward the request within 24 hours after the request is submitted delays the running of the 30-day advance notice period until the request has been forwarded.

An emergency discharge or transfer may be implemented as necessary pursuant to state or federal law during the period of time a hearing decision is rendered. Notice of an emergency discharge or transfer to the resident, the resident's legal guardian or representative, and the local ombudsman council, if requested by the patient, must be by telephone or in person. The notice must be given before the transfer, if possible, or as soon thereafter as practicable. A district ombudsman council conducting a review under this subsection must do so within 24 hours after receipt of the request.

Resident's Rights

According to Florida state statute, all licensees of nursing home facilities must adopt and make public a statement of the rights and responsibilities of the residents that assures each resident of the following:

1. the right to civil and religious liberties
2. the right to private and uncensored communication
3. the right of access to the resident by individuals providing health, social, and legal services and the right of the resident to deny access to such individuals
4. the right to present grievances on his or her own behalf
5. the right to organize and participate in resident groups
6. the right to participate in social, religious, and community activities that do not interfere with the rights of other residents
7. the right to examine the results of the most recent inspection of the facility
8. the right to manage his or her own financial affairs
9. the right to be fully informed of services available in the facility and of related charges for such services
10. the right to be informed of his or her medical condition and proposed treatment
11. the right to refuse medication or treatment and to be informed of the consequences of such decisions
12. the right to receive adequate and appropriate health care and protective and support services
13. the right to have privacy in treatment and in caring for personal needs
14. the right to be treated courteously, fairly, and with the fullest measure of dignity
15. the right to be free from mental and physical abuse
16. the right to be transferred or discharged only for medical reasons
17. the right to freedom of choice in selecting a personal physician
18. the right to retain and use personal clothing and possessions

19. the right to have copies of the rules and regulations of the facility

20. the right to receive notice before the room of the resident is changed

21. the right to be informed of the bed reservation policy for a hospitalization for residents of Medicaid-certified or Medicare-certified facilities

22. the right to challenge a decision by the facility to discharge or transfer the resident

Any resident whose rights are deprived or infringed upon has a cause of action against any licensee responsible for the violation. The action may be brought by the resident, by his or her guardian, by a person or organization acting on behalf of the resident with the consent of the resident or his or her guardian, or by the personal representative of the estate of a deceased resident when the cause of death resulted from the deprivation or infringement of the decedent's rights.

Office of the Local Long-Term Care Ombudsman

The purpose of the Office of the Local Long-Term Care Ombudsman is to identify, investigate, and resolve complaints made by or on behalf of residents of long-term care facilities, relating to public or private agencies, guardians, or representative payees that may adversely affect the health, safety, welfare, or rights of the residents.

Selecting a Nursing Home

It is important to first define the goal for the patient for whom care will be given. For instance, how long will he or she need to remain a resident? Is he or she expected to recover to the degree that long-term residency is not necessary? The nursing home conducts an assessment of the resident's need and develops a plan of care. The Health Care Financing Administration (HCFA), which administers the Medicaid and Medicare programs at the federal level, requires facilities to review all aspects of the resident's needs. Staff members will be involved, during which time both the patient and family may also participate.

Florida's Agency for Health Care Administration is charged with providing information to the public about all the licensed nursing home facilities operating in this state. This information provides consumer-friendly printed and electronic formats to assist consumers and their families in comparing and evaluating nursing home facilities. There is now an Internet site and printed material which contain relevant information about each nursing home facility in this state. Each nursing home's licensure status and rating history for the past 5 years is included. This information can be found on the Internet at www.medicare.gov. The viewer should click on Nursing Home Compare.

CHAPTER 18

ELDER ABUSE

Many elderly persons in Florida are presently suffering from the infirmities of aging that are caused by organic brain damage, or other physical, mental, or emotional illnesses. Often, an elderly person's ability to adequately provide for his or her own care or protection is impaired due to these infirmities. Unfortunately, there are those who by deception or intimidation obtain, or attempt to obtain, assets from such infirmed elderly persons. There are also times when a caregiver will intentionally refuse to provide an infirmed elderly person with the care, supervision and services necessary to maintain the elderly person's physical and mental health, including food, clothing, medicine, shelter and medical care.

Fortunately, the Florida legislature has recognized the need to provide for the detection and correction of such abuse, neglect and exploitation of the elderly and disabled adults. The legislature has addressed this need by establishing the Adult Protective Services Act.

These laws require the Department of Children and Families to conduct an investigation of all reports received that allege abuse, neglect, or exploitation of an elderly person or a disabled adult. The purpose of the Department's investigation is to determine if there is evidence that a victim has been abused, neglected, or exploited and if assistance is necessary to protect the individual's health and safety.

This statute requires the Department of Children and Families to establish and maintain a central abuse registry and tracking system for all such reports made in writing or through a statewide toll-free telephone number. Any person may use the statewide toll-free telephone number to report known or suspected abuse, neglect, or exploitation of an elderly person or a disabled adult at any hour of the day or night, any day of the week. This toll free telephone number is 1-800-96ABUSE (1-800-962-2873). All records concerning reports of abuse, neglect, or exploitation made to this registry and tracking system are confidential and may not be disclosed.

The Adult Protective Services Act states that it is mandatory for any person, including but not limited to, physicians, hospital personnel, mental health professionals, nursing home or assisted living facility staff, law enforcement officers and bank employees who know or have reasonable cause to suspect an elderly person or disabled person is being abused, neglected or exploited to immediately report such knowledge or suspicion to the central abuse registry and tracking system on the state-wide toll-free number. The statute further provides that any person who makes such a report or participates in a judicial proceeding resulting therefrom is presumed to be acting in good faith and is immune from any civil or criminal liability, unless a lack of good faith is shown. A person who knowingly and willfully fails to report a case of known or suspected abuse, neglect, or exploitation of an elderly person or disabled adult or who prevents another person from doing so commits a second degree misdemeanor which is punishable by up to sixty days in jail and a fine of up to $500. Likewise, a person who knowingly and willfully makes a false report of abuse, neglect, or exploitation, or who advises another to make a false report, commits a second-degree misdemeanor.

Upon receiving an oral or written report of known or suspected abuse, neglect or exploitation of an elderly person or disabled adult, the central abuse registry and tracking system must determine if the report requires an immediate protective service investigation. If the report requires an immediate investigation, the Department's designated adult protective investigator responsible for protective investigations will be notified to ensure the prompt initiation of an investigation. For reports not requiring an immediate protective service investigation, the Department's district staff will be notified in sufficient time to allow for an investigation to be commenced within 24 hours.

A protective service investigator will visit the alleged victim within 24 hours of receiving a report of abuse, neglect or exploitation of an elderly person or a disabled adult. If a report of abuse or neglect is made on the weekend or a holiday, the investigator will still make an initial visit to the alleged victim within 24 hours. However, if the report made on the weekend or a holiday relates to an allegation of exploitation, the investigator will not make the initial visit until the next working day.

The protective service investigator will, during his or her initial visit, interview the alleged victim and all persons who have knowledge of the situation. The protective service investigator will then determine whether there is an indication that an elderly person or a disabled adult is being abused, neglected or exploited. The investigator will also determine if there is any harm or threatened harm to the elderly person or the disabled adult, the nature and extent of the injuries, abuse or neglect, and determine the person responsible. Of special importance is the fact that the protective service investigator will also determine the protection, treatment and other services necessary to safeguard and insure the elderly or disabled person's well-being and cause the delivery of those services. The Department may, with the consent of the elderly person or the disabled adult, cause that person to be referred to a licensed physician or an emergency department in a hospital for medical examination and diagnosis or treatment if areas of trauma are visible or the person complains of, or otherwise exhibits signs or symptoms indicating of, a need for medical attention which is the consequence of the suspected abuse or neglect.

If the protective service investigator has reasonable cause to believe the elderly or disabled person is suffering from abuse or neglect that presents a risk of death or serious physical injury and that elderly or disabled person lacks the capacity to consent to emergency protective services, the Department of Children and Families may transport this person to a medical or protective service facility for treatment. The Department must file a petition with the Circuit Court and demonstrate by clear and convincing evidence that the emergency protective services should continue. If an order to continue emergency services is issued by the Circuit Judge, it must state the services to be provided and designate an individual or agency to be responsible for performing essential services on behalf of the elderly person or disabled adult.

No later than thirty days after receiving the initial report, the Department of Children and Families shall complete its investigation and classify the report as confirmed or unfounded, or else close the report without classification. A person who is named as a perpetrator in a confirmed report of abuse, neglect, or exploitation of a disabled adult or elderly person is subject to a civil penalty of $250 for the first offense, $500 for the second offense and $1,000 for the third and subsequent offenses. A disabled adult or an elderly person who has been named as a victim in a confirmed report of abuse, neglect or exploitation has a cause of action against any perpetrator named in the confirmed report and may recover actual and punitive damages for such abuse, neglect and exploitation.

With respect to any case of reported abuse, neglect, or exploitation of an elderly person or disabled adult, the Department, when appropriate, shall transmit all reports received by it which pertain to the investigation to the state attorney of the circuit where the incident occurred. The state attorney is authorized by Florida statute to criminally prosecute a person who is determined to have knowingly abused, neglected or exploited an elderly or disabled person. A person convicted of abusing, neglecting or exploiting an elderly or disabled adult person will be guilty of a felony of the third degree that is punishable by up to five years in prison and a fine of up to $5,000. A person convicted of aggravated abuse or neglect of an elderly or disabled adult person will be guilty of a felony of the second degree that is punishable by up to fifteen years in prison and a fine of up to $10,000. If the funds, assets or property involved in the exploitation of the elderly or disabled adult person are valued at $100,000 or more, the convicted offender commits a felony of the first degree which is punishable by up to thirty years in prison and a fine of up to $10,000.

In 2014, the Florida Legislature amended chapter 825, Florida Statutes, to expand the definition of exploitation of the elderly. Exploitation now includes the breach of a fiduciary duty by an individual trustee that causes an "unauthorized appropriation." Previous versions of the statute only covered breaches by a guardian or agent under a power of attorney. The amendment added definitions of "unauthorized appropriation." For individual trustees and guardians, "unauthorized appropriation" is defined as (1) fraud in obtaining appointment; (2) abuse of power; or, (3) waste, embezzlement, or intentional mismanagement of assets. For an agent under a power of attorney, "unauthorized appropriation" is defined as (1) fraud in obtaining appointment; (2) abuse of power; (3) waste, embezzlement, or intentional mismanagement of assets; or, (4) actions contrary to the principal's sole benefit or best interest. Exploitation was also expanded to include misappropriation of funds owned by an elderly person from a personal account, joint account, or convenience account. Exploitation was further defined to include intentional or negligent failure to use an elderly person's income and assets for necessities for the elderly person's support and maintenance by a caregiver or person in a position of trust with the elderly person.

CHAPTER 19

MEDICAID NURSING HOME ASSISTANCE

- Eligibility
- Non-Countable Assets
- Lady Bird Deed
- Transferring Assets
- Promissory Notes, Loans and Mortgages
- Undue Hardship
- Irrevocable Annuities
- Half-A-Loaf
- Personal Service Contract
- Exemptions to the Transfer Rules
- Supplemental Needs Trusts and Pooled Trusts
- Assisted Living Facility Medicaid Waiver Program
- Medicaid Estate Recovery
- Medicaid Managed Care
- Just Say No

Eligibility

A nursing home patient may be eligible for assistance in paying a portion of his or her skilled or custodial nursing home cost through the state of Florida's institutional care program. However, there is a maximum amount of countable assets that a person applying for assistance and his or her spouse can own and still receive assistance. The institutionalized spouse entering a nursing home cannot own more than $2,000 in countable assets. In the year 2015, the community spouse who is not residing in the nursing home can not own more than $119,220 in countable assets. A person who has no spouse can only retain $2,000 in countable assets. However, a person with an income of less than $856 per month can have assets of $5,000.

There is also a maximum amount of monthly income that the institutionalized spouse can receive and still be eligible for nursing home assistance. The monthly gross income available to the institutionalized spouse cannot exceed the state monthly income cap of $2,199 in 2015. However, a nursing home patient with a gross monthly income in excess of $2,199 for 2015 can still qualify for the institutional care program by establishing an irrevocable qualified income trust. This trust is often referred to as a Miller Trust, after the name of the Colorado case that originally approved this concept. The nursing home patient's income in excess of $2,199 is irrevocably assigned to the irrevocable qualified income trust that is used to pay the patient's medical and nursing home expenses.

In determining the institutionalized spouse's income available to pay the cost of the nursing home, a community spouse is first permitted to retain a minimum monthly maintenance income needs allowance that is sometimes referred to as a MMMNIA. This means that the community spouse may retain his or her income plus the portion of the institutionalized spouse's income necessary to allow the community spouse $1,966.25 in income per month. There may be an additional amount of income diverted from the institutionalized spouse if the community spouse can demonstrate excess shelter expenses. This amount will increase on July 1, 2015.

Non-Countable Assets

All assets owned by the institutionalized spouse or by the non-institutionalized spouse are considered countable assets unless exempted by state regulation. An individual with an equity interest in his or her home in excess of $552,000 is not eligible for long-term care. Home equity is calculated using the current market value of the home minus any debt. The current market value is the amount for which it can be reasonably expected to sell on the open market in the geographic area. If the home is held in any form of shared ownership, only the fractional interest of the person requesting long-term care assistance should be considered. The home equity policy does not apply if the residence is being occupied by the nursing home resident's spouse, a child under age 21, or a blind or disabled child is living in the residence. The home equity must be revalued each year that the applicant remains on Medicaid nursing home assistance. This home equity limitation may be waived when a denial of long-term care eligibility will result in a demonstrated hardship to the individual.

One vehicle is excluded in computing countable assets regardless of its age or value. A second vehicle is generally excluded if it is more than seven years old. If the total face value of the patient's whole life insurance policies is $2,500 or less, the cash value of the policies is excluded as an asset. The full value of an irrevocable burial contract is excluded as an asset. Likewise, there is a $2,500 exclusion for bank accounts that have been designated for burial expenses.

It is also important to consider the exemptions and maximum allowances for tangible personal property such as clothing, jewelry, tools of a trade, pets, and household goods such as furniture and appliances. A community spouse is entitled to exclude all personal property, if his or her spouse is in a nursing home. A single person may exclude a wedding ring, one engagement ring, and any items required because of the individual's medical or physical condition. A single person may also exclude household goods and personal effects up to a value of $2,000. It will be assumed that the household goods and personal effects are less than $2,000, unless the individual applying for personal assistance indicates he or she owns items of unusual value.

The total value of an individual retirement account (IRA) owned by an institutionalized spouse is not counted as an available asset if it is placed into payment status over the life expectancy of the institutionalized spouse. Likewise, the total value of an individual retirement account (IRA) owned by a community spouse is not counted as an available asset if it is placed into payment status over the life expectancy of the community spouse. Most districts of the Department of Children and Families require the IRA payments to be paid over Social Security's life expectancy tables. Other districts require the payments to be paid over the Social Security Administration's life expectancy tables.

LIFE SITUATION #10

George has been in a nursing home for over twenty days. He will need to remain there because a massive stroke has disabled him to the degree that he will no longer be able to perform his daily living activities. George and his wife, Helen, own a residence having a fair market value of $250,000, and $139,220 in savings, and a 2005 car with over 150,000 miles. George's monthly income is $1,000 from Social Security and $1,500 from a pension. Helen receives $700 each month from Social Security. Since a community spouse (the spouse living outside the nursing home) can only own $119,220 in countable assets and a nursing home spouse can only own $2,000 in countable assets in 2015, George is presently not eligible for Medicaid nursing assistance. One way to obtain eligibility is for Helen to replace the 2005 automobile with a new one that will cost about $20,000. This purchase will not disqualify George from Medicaid assistance since something of value was received by Helen and the new automobile is a non-countable asset. Since George's income exceeds the 2015 monthly income cap of $2,199, he will need to establish a Qualified Income Trust (QIT). The trust will need to state that any monthly income over the monthly income cap of $2,199 is assigned to the trustee of the trust. The excess income of $401 per month that is paid to the QIT will be used for George's care. Helen is entitled to a minimum monthly maintenance income needs allowance in 2015 of at least $1,966.25 each month and can divert

$1,266.25 of George's income ($1,966.25 minus Helen's $700 Social Security) to meet her living needs. George will be able to retain $105 each month for his personal needs allowance. George's remaining income of $1,129 after Helen receives her minimum monthly maintenance income needs allowance and George receives his $105 personal needs allowance becomes George's patient pay responsibility to the nursing home. The additional monthly cost of the nursing home will be paid to the nursing home facility by the state of Florida's Department of Children and Families.

Lady Bird Deed

A life estate deed permits the present owner of real property to retain the use and enjoyment of the real property during the remaining lifetime of the owner while presently conveying the remainder interest at the death of the present owner to another person. Upon the death of the owner, the real property is automatically the real property of the person who received the remainder interest. No probate is required on the death of the present owner because the real property has already been conveyed during the lifetime of the present owner to the person who receives the remainder interest. Normally, a conveyance of a life estate results in a gift of the remainder interest and the person conveying the remainder interest must timely file a federal gift tax return if the fair market value of the remainder interest exceeds the annual gift tax exclusion amount which is presently $14,000. In addition, the owner of the life estate must obtain the joinder of the owner of the remainder interest in order to convey this real property to a third person during lifetime.

There is another form of life estate deed known as a "Lady Bird Deed," that permits the owner of the real property to retain the use and enjoyment of the real property during his or her lifetime, but to also divest the remainder man of his or her remainder interest without his or her joinder or consent. A Lady Bird deed permits the owner of the life estate to still convey or mortgage the real property to a third person. In addition, there is no gift tax return required despite remainder interest having a fair market value exceeding the federal gift tax exclusion that is presently $14,000. This is important because the Department of Children and Families will not find that a gift of any interest in real property has been made if the remainder interest is granted by a Lady Bird Deed interest and the real property conveyed by Lady Bird deed will still be considered the homestead of the owner of the life estate if he or she is residing there. Also, a judgment against the remainder man will not attach to the real property described in the lady bird deed during the lifetime of the holder of the life estate. There will still be a full "stepped-up" basis in the real property when the life tenant dies.

In order to establish a Lady Bird deed, the present owner must state in that deed that the present owner, as the grantor, is retaining a life estate, without any liability for waste, and with the full power and authority in said life tenant to sell, convey, mortgage, lease or otherwise manage and dispose of the property described therein, in fee simple, with or without consideration, without joinder of the remainder man, and with full power and authority to retain any and all proceeds generated thereby, and upon the death of the last life tenant, the remainder, if any, passes to a certain person as the grantee.

It is important to understand that if the remainder man predeceases the grantor, then upon the death of the grantor, the real property passes to the remainder man's estate.

Transferring Assets

A gift to someone other than a spouse or a minor child or disabled child may cause the donor and his or her spouse to be ineligible for nursing home assistance for a period of time. Transfers made before November 1, 2007, to someone other than a spouse or a minor child or a disabled child for no consideration caused the nursing home patient to be ineligible for Medicaid assistance for a certain period determined by dividing the amount of the uncompensated transfer by the state determined average cost of nursing home care. Thus, a gift by the nursing home patient to someone other than a spouse or a minor child or a disabled child in October of 2007, results in an ineligibility period lasting for 10 months beginning with the month in which the gift was made.

Transfers made on or after November 1, 2007, to someone other than a spouse or a minor child or a disabled child for no consideration will cause the nursing home patient to be ineligible for Medicaid assistance on the later of the following dates:

(1) The first day the individual would be eligible for long-term care Medicaid were it not for imposition of the transfer period (this includes the filing of an application and meeting all other program criteria for long term care Medicaid), or (2) the first day of the month in which the individual transfers the assets, or (3) the first day following the end of an existing penalty period.

Thus, a gift by a person to someone other than a spouse or a minor child or a disabled child of $79,950 in November of 2013, who then enters the nursing home on April 15, 2015 with less than $2,000, will result in an ineligibility period lasting for 10 months beginning May 1, 2015, which is the first month after an application is filed and the person meets all other program criteria for long term care Medicaid. This means that the applicant who made the gift of $79,950 in November of 2013 will not be eligible for Medicaid nursing home assistance until March, 2016. This is because the average cost of a nursing home in Florida is $7,995. The look-back period for gifts is 60 months. Since the gift was made to someone other than a spouse or a minor child or a disabled child within the look-back period of 60 months from entry into the nursing home, the ineligibility period is 10 months from the month after entry into the nursing home. There is no fine of penalty if the recipient of the gift repays the gift to the nursing home patient who then uses the funds to pay for his or her nursing care.

Promissory Notes, Loans and Mortgages

All promissory notes, loans and mortgages signed on or after November 1, 2007, will be considered a transfer of assets without fair compensation, unless the promissory note, loan or mortgage has a repayment term that is actuarially sound based on Social Security's life expectancy tables, and has payments made in equal amounts during the term of the loan with no deferral or balloon payments and the note does not allow for debt forgiveness.

Undue Hardship

A nursing home patient who has made an uncompensated transfer subjecting him or her to a penalty period affecting eligibility and a person with a home equity interest exceeding $552,000 must be offered an opportunity by the Department of Children and Families to demonstrate that the imposition of the penalty period will create an undue hardship. This opportunity must be granted before the disposition of the application. Nursing home facilities are allowed to apply for an undue hardship waiver on behalf of an individual with the consent of the applicant or the designated representative. An undue hardship exists when application of the transfer of asset penalty or excess home equity penalty will deprive the nursing home patient of medical care such that his or her health or life would be endangered, or the individual will be deprived of food, clothing, shelter or other necessities of life.

Other federal and state laws prohibit a nursing home from evicting a resident without transferring the person to a safe place. Thus, the nursing home might be required to continue to provide care to an indigent patient without receiving public assistance until the undue hardship waiver has been determined.

Irrevocable Annuities

When an individual purchases an annuity, he or she generally pays to the insurance company that issues the annuity a lump sum of money, in return for which he or she is promised regular payments of income in certain amounts. The payments may continue for a fixed period of time (for example 10 years) or for as long as the individual (or another designated beneficiary) lives, thus creating an ongoing income stream. The annuity may or may not include a remainder clause stating that if the person who owns the annuity dies, the insurance company converts whatever is remaining in the annuity into a lump sum and pays it to a designated beneficiary.

Annuities, although usually purchased to provide a source of income for retirement, are occasionally used in conjunction with Medicaid planning. To avoid penalizing persons who validly purchased annuities as part of a retirement plan, but to capture those annuities that were purchased to shelter assets, a determination is made by the Department of Children and Families that the return to the annuitant is fairly computed. If the expected return on the annuity is commensurate with a reasonable estimate of the life expectancy of the beneficiary, the annuity is deemed sound for actuarial purposes and is not considered to have been purchased to shelter assets. The annuity must also be irrevocable and non-assignable. The periodic payments (including the interest portion) are counted as unearned income in the eligibility determination and patient responsibility. An annuity that is revocable or non-assignable is not considered a countable asset. If the annuity is revocable, the asset value is the amount the purchaser would receive from the annuity insurer if the annuity is cancelled. If the annuity is assignable, the asset value is the amount the annuity can be sold for on the secondary market.

To determine that an annuity is sound for actuarial purposes, the life expectancy tables, compiled from information published by the Office of the Actuary of the Social Security Administration, are used. The average number of years of expected life remaining for the individual must coincide with the length of the annuity. If the individual is not reasonably expected to live longer than the guarantee period of the annuity, the individual will not receive fair market value for the annuity based on the projected return. In this case, the annuity is not actuarially sound and a transfer of assets for less than fair market value has taken place, possibly subjecting the individual to a penalty. The penalty is assessed based on a transfer of assets for less than fair market value that is considered to have occurred at the time the annuity was purchased. For example, a male at age 65 has a life expectancy of 14.96 years according to the table. Thus, if he purchases a $14,080 annuity to be paid over the course of 10 years, the annuity is actuarially sound. However, a male at age 80 has a life expectancy of only 6.98 years. Thus, if he purchases an annuity to be paid over 10 years, the amount that will be received for the last 3 years is considered a transfer of assets for less than fair market value, and that amount is subject to penalty.

The new Medicaid laws still permit a spouse with countable assets in excess of the $119,220 community spouse resource allowance to purchase an annuity with the excess assets. The annuity must be paid to the community spouse over no longer than his or her life expectancy. However, the new law requires that the state be named the first beneficiary for at least the total amount of medical assistance paid on behalf of the annuitant, except when the owner of the annuity has a spouse, minor or disabled child. In this case, the State of Florida may be named as the secondary beneficiary after the spouse, minor or disabled child. Since the new law addresses only the medical assistance paid on behalf of the person over whose life the payments are to be made, there is a question as to whether there is a repayment obligation if the annuitant is the community spouse.

Half-A-Loaf

There is a method used to shorten the delay that a single person will otherwise experience in attaining Medicaid nursing home assistance by gifting countable assets. It is commonly referred to as "half-a-loaf." The single person will give a portion of his or her assets to his or her children and purchase a Medicaid qualifying annuity with the remaining balance of his or her countable assets. The Department of Children and Families will determine the single person to be ineligible for nursing home assistance for the amount of the gift divided by the average cost of a nursing home that is $7,995 per month. However, the cost of the nursing home during the ineligible period will be paid by the Medicaid Qualifying annuity's monthly payment. By example, Mrs. Jones who is a widow owns $125,000 and receives Social Security of $1,500 per month. If Mrs. Jones needs custodial nursing care, she could give her children $65,000. This will disqualify her for Medicaid nursing home assistance for 9 months ($65,000 divided by $7,995 = 8.13 months that is rounded up to 9 months). If the average cost of the nursing home is $8,000 and she receives $1,500 per month, she will need $58,500 to pay the nursing home the remaining balance of $6,500 per month for nine months. She could purchase before entering the nursing home an irrevocable annuity for $58,500 that will pay her Qualified Income Trust $6,500 per month for 9 months and she can retain $1,500 that is less than her $2,000 resource allowance. If Mrs. Jones dies within the nine months, the remaining annuity payments will be paid to her beneficiary named in the annuity, since the Department of Children and Family never paid anything toward her care. This Medicaid Compliant annuity must be irrevocable, non-assignable, structured with an actuarially sound payout, providing equal monthly payments, naming the Department of Children and Families as the primary beneficiary.

Personal Service Contract

Of great concern to a senior citizen is the right to continue to live at home despite the need for assistance and personalized care. Another concern is that there will be someone to advocate for him or her in the event of incapacity and the level of care increases or placement in a nursing home becomes necessary.

The assistance necessary to keep a person at home, and not in a nursing home, is often provided at no cost by a child, another family member or a friend. A subsequent reimbursement to a family member or friend who has spent months and perhaps years providing the care and assistance necessary to keep the senior at home may result in denial of Medicaid nursing assistance to this senior citizen. This is because an individual who makes an uncompensated transfer of assets within the look-back period for Medicaid assistance will be presumed to have made a disqualifying gift.

A period of Medicaid ineligibility will usually not result if the person in need of assistance initially contracts with a family member or a friend before these personal services are rendered. In such event, real or personal property estimated to equal the value of the services to be rendered to the infirmed person can be transferred in exchange for an agreement to provide the personal services over the infirmed person's lifetime. There is no disqualifying gift in this instance because the personal service contract provides that the infirmed person will receive services having a value equal to the property being transferred.

The personal service agreement must be in the form of a binding written contract that is signed by both parties. The contract should state that the services are to be provided solely by the caregiver and that these services cannot be delegated to another person. This contract should state that the services will be provided to the infirmed person as needed. The contract should recognize that the need for certain services will increase or decrease with time. At a minimum, the contract should confirm that the family member or friend will monitor the infirmed person's health care, secure necessary health care, provide financial management and visit the person to provide the services on a periodic basis.

A personal service contract's term is most often for the infirmed person's life expectancy. This is necessary to avoid a concern that the person is not receiving sufficient care in return for his or her payment and that a gift is being made.

The method used to determine the maximum amount of real or personal property to be transferred in exchange for the promise of lifetime personal care is to multiply the reasonable wage in the community for these services times the number of hours per week reasonably expected of the caregiver times the 52 weeks in the year times the infirm person's life expectancy, which is determined from the Health Care Financing Administration's life expectancy charts.

It is important to remember that the person who agrees to provide the personal services will have to report, as income, any payment received or the value of any property received as a result of the contract. Also, the infirmed person who will be receiving the services may recognize a capital gain for income tax purposes when his or her assets are transferred in exchange for the personal services to be provided. The advice of a certified public accountant and an attorney before entering into a personal service agreement is recommended.

Exemptions to the Transfer Rules

Transfers to a spouse or to another person for the sole benefit of the spouse, or transfers from a spouse to another person for the sole benefit of the spouse are exempt from transfer penalties. Transfers to a disabled child or to a trust established solely for the benefit of a disabled child are also exempt in determining the transfer penalties. The transfer penalties do not apply to transfers to a trust established solely for the benefit of a disabled individual under age 65.

A transfer of an individual's home is exempt if the recipient is the spouse, a child who is blind, disabled, or under age 21, a child who had resided at the individual's home for two years prior to the institutionalization and had cared for the parent-applicant or a sibling with an equity interest who had resided there for one year prior to the institutionalization.

An applicant is considered to have established a non-countable trust for Medicaid purposes if his or her assets were used to form all or part of the assets of the trust and if any of the following persons established such a trust other than by will: the applicant, the applicant's spouse, a person (including a court or administrative body) with legal authority to act in place of or on behalf of the individual or the applicant's spouse, or a person (including any court or administrative body) acting upon the direction or request of the applicant or the applicant's spouse.

If the trust includes assets of an individual and assets of another person or persons as noted above, the trust will be considered to have been established by the individual to the extent of the portion comprising the individual's assets.

In the case of revocable trusts, the assets owned by the trust are considered a resource available to the person applying for Medicaid, and payments to or for the benefit of the applicant will be considered income of the applicant. Any other payment from the trust (presumably payments to third persons) will be considered assets disposed of by the applicant and falling under the rules governing the transfer of assets (subject to the 60-month lookback period).

With an irrevocable trust, if there are any circumstances under which payment from the trust could be made to or for the benefit of the applicant, the portion of the assets of the trust or the income from which payment is made to the applicant will be considered resources available to the applicant. Payments from that portion of assets of the trust or income paid to or for the benefit of the individual will be considered a transfer of assets.

Supplemental Needs Trusts and Pooled Trusts

Individuals with mental and physical disabilities often lack the ability to support themselves due to the inability to work full-time on a recurring basis. Government benefits such as Supplemental Security Income (SSI) and Medicaid will help pay for a disabled person's basic needs and medical care if he or she does not receive sufficient income and does not have sufficient assets to pay for these costs.

The maximum monthly countable income that a person can receive and be eligible for SSI benefits is $733 in 2015. In Florida, a person who is eligible for SSI benefits automatically receives Medicaid.

If the disabled person meets the income and asset guidelines, Medicaid pays for the cost of health care provided by physicians, hospitals, pharmacists and other health care providers. SSI may also pay for training programs.

Unearned income received from other benefit payments, financial gifts, annuity payments and payments from a trust fund paid directly to the SSI recipient reduces his or her monthly SSI payment dollar for dollar. Earned income is also counted but treated differently.

In calculating countable income, there is a general $20 disregard applied to most incomes. In calculating the earned income offset to SSI, the first $65 per month of earned income and one-half of the remaining work-related income is not counted. The remaining one-half of work-related income will be counted against a person's SSI benefit. Payments made by another person for a recipient's food and shelter reduces the SSI benefit up to a maximum of $278.55 per month in 2015.

The asset limit for an SSI recipient is $2,000. Anything that can be converted to cash will be considered toward this $2,000 limit. This includes bank accounts, 401(k) benefits, cash values in some life insurance policies and trust funds where the trustee has the discretion to pay for the recipient's support. A homestead, one car and some personal effects are not counted as assets. The asset limit for Medicaid only is $5,000.

If a trust is established to provide for the basic support needs such as housing and food, the recipient will be denied SSI because the trust assets in excess of $2,000 will be considered available to the recipient. A person applying for Medicaid only will be denied Medicaid assistance if his or her trust assets exceed $5,000. It is possible for a trust fund to be created to provide supplemental services to a disabled person without depriving the recipient of SSI and Medicaid benefits. The assets of the trust will not be counted if the terms of the trust agreement state that the trust funds are not to be expended for basic needs that are provided by SSI, but are only to supplement these benefits.

A Supplemental Needs Trust authorizes the trustee to pay only the expenses of goods and services that are supplemental to the beneficiary's basic needs (food and shelter). Food and shelter expenses cannot be covered by the trust. Some examples of allowable expenses that can be paid from a Supplemental Needs Trust are medical equipment not covered by Medicaid; medical, nursing and dental care, tests not covered by another source; insurance premiums (Health, Dental, Life, Car, and Renter); clothing, personal assistance; private counseling or case management; guardianship and advocacy services; computer hardware and software; school or camp tuition; home appliances; furniture; telephone and internet charges.

Some of the charges that are not allowable to be paid from a supplemental needs trust are food and groceries; rent and mortgage payments; property taxes; condominium fees and utility charges.

The beneficiary of a special needs trust (also known as supplemental needs trust) must be an individual under 65 years of age who is determined disabled by the Social Security Administration. This means the beneficiary who is unable to engage in substantial gainful activity by reason of any medically determinable physical or mental impairment that can be expected to result in death, or which has lasted or can be expected to last for a continuous period of not less than twelve months.

A special needs trust is one that is established for the disabled person's benefit by a parent, grandparent, legal guardian or the court with money due to the disabled beneficiary. The state paying the Medicaid benefits for a disabled person will receive all amounts remaining in the trust upon the death of the individual, up to an amount equal to the total medical assistance paid on behalf of the individual under a State plan. Court approval is not required and there need not be a pay-back provision in a trust created by a third party such as a grandparent.

Another type of trust can be established for the special needs of a disabled person without the assets being considered available. This is called a pooled trust. It is managed by a non-profit organization that pools the funds of that trust with the funds from all participants. However, there is a separate sub account for each beneficiary. A pooled income trust can be established for a disabled person, regardless of his or her age. At the beneficiary's death, the amount remaining in the beneficiary's account is paid to the state that provided the Medicaid assistance to the total amount of benefits provided. However, the remaining assets can be left in the pooled trust for other disabled persons and no payback is required.

Assisted Living Facility Medicaid Waiver Program

The State of Florida's Assisted Living Medicaid Waiver Program pays for services provided to financially and physically eligible residents of assisted living facilities who would otherwise need placement in a nursing home. Some of the services covered under the Assisted Living Facility Medicaid Waiver Program include case management, personal care services, medication management, administration, intermittent nursing care services, occupational therapy, physical therapy, speech therapy, therapeutic social and recreational services, specialized medical equipment and incontinence supplies.

The rules governing the Assisted Living Waiver Medicaid Program changed as of July 1, 2003. This change is intended to align the Assisted Living Waiver Programs rules involving asset allocations and income allowances to spouses and dependents with the current Medicaid nursing home institutional care program.

For persons applying for this assistance, the change affects the amount of assets the applicant and his or her spouse can own and still qualify for this program. Previously, only the assets of the person applying for the assisted living waiver were considered. The new policy requires that all countable resources owned solely by either the applicant or his or her spouse and the resources owned jointly by a married couple are considered in determining eligibility. Those countable assets that exceed the patient's allowable resource limit of $2,000, and the 2015 community spouse's resource limit of $119,220, will be considered available to the spouse applying for the Assisted Living Waiver Program. Thus, the husband and wife having countable assets in 2015 in excess of $121,270, will have to spend down the countable assets to the allowable amount before the spouse will be eligible for the Assisted Living Waiver Medicaid Program.

The resident applying for a Medicaid Assisted Living Waiver must be residing in an assisted living facility that is certified as a Medicaid provider and have a contract with the Department of Elder Affairs. The assisted living facility must provide semi-private rooms and bathrooms and also have an extended congregate care (ECC) or limited nursing service (LNS) license. A person residing in an assisted living facility applying for an Assisted Living Medicaid Waiver must be 65 or older, or be age 60 to 65 and be determined disabled according to the Social Security standards. This person must also meet the nursing facility level-of-care criteria as determined by the Florida Department of Elder Affairs CARES team. This means the resident must require assistance with four or more activities of daily living (ADLs); or require assistance with three ADLs plus assistance with the administration of medication; or require total help with one or more ADLs; or have a diagnosis of Alzheimer Disease or another type of dementia and require assistance with two or more ADLs; or have a diagnosis of a degenerative or chronic medical condition requiring nursing services that cannot be provided in a standard licensed ALF but are available for an ALF licensed to provide limited nursing services; or extended congregate care services; or be a Medicaid-eligible resident awaiting discharge from a nursing home who cannot return to a private residence because of the need for supervision, personal care services, periodic nursing services or a combination of the three; and who is receiving case management and in need of assisted living services as determined by the community case manager and determined to meet eligibility criteria by CARES.

Regardless of the facility's license status, residents living in an Assisted Living Facility cannot have conditions that require 24-hour nursing supervision. The only exception is for a resident who is receiving hospice services from a licensed hospice while continuing to reside in an Assisted Living Facility.

Medicaid Estate Recovery

The 1999 Florida Legislature passed the Medicaid Estate Recovery Act. The legislature stated that its intent in passing this law is to supplement Medicaid funds that are used to provide medical services to eligible persons. Medicaid estate recovery is to be accomplished through the filing of claims against the estate of deceased Medicaid recipients. A recent Florida statute states that the personal representative (executor) of the estate of the decedent must serve Florida's Agency for Health Care Administration with a copy of the notice to creditors within 3 months after the first publication of the notice of creditors. The claim amount is calculated as the total amount paid to or for the benefit of the recipient for medical assistance on behalf of the recipient after he or she reached age 55 years of age. There is no claim against estates of recipients who had not yet reached age 55 years of age.

This statute confirms that the claim for Medicaid funds will not be enforced if the Medicaid recipient is survived by:
1. A spouse;
2. A child or children under 21 years of age; or
3. A child or children who are blind or permanently and totally disabled pursuant to the eligibility requirements of the Social Security Act.

This statute also clarifies that in accordance with the Florida Constitution, no claim will be enforced against any property that is determined to be the homestead of the deceased Medicaid recipient and is determined by court order to be exempt from the claims of creditors of the deceased Medicaid recipient.

The statute further states that the Agency for Health Care Administration is not to recover from an estate if doing so would cause an undue hardship for the heirs. The hardship to be considered by the agency in reviewing a hardship request is whether the heir:
1. Currently resides in the residence of the deceased;
2. Resided in the residence of the deceased at the time of the death of the deceased;
3. Made the residence his or her primary residence for the 12 months immediately preceding the death of the deceased; and
4. Owns another residence.

Other factors which will be considered are whether the heir would be deprived of food, clothing, shelter, or medical care necessary for the maintenance of life or health. Another factor will be whether the heir can document that he or she provided full-time care to the recipient which delayed the recipient's entry into a nursing home. In such event, the heir must be either the decedent's sibling or the son or daughter of the decedent and must have resided with the recipient for at least 1 year prior to the recipient's death. Another factor is whether the cost involved in the sale will be equal to, or exceed, the value of the property.

Medicaid Managed Care

Beginning in 2014, a statewide system of Medicaid Managed Care requires current and future Medicaid recipients to enroll in a Managed Care Plan that is administered by a Managed Care Organization (MCO). Each long term care Plan is required to offer, at a minimum, coverage of certain health care services that are vital to the Medicaid recipient's needs.

Although there are seven MCO's that operate in Florida, each region may contain only a few. In Citrus and Hernando Counties, only American Elder Care, Sunshine State Health Plan, and United Healthcare offer plans. In Pasco County, Molina Healthcare will offer a Plan in addition to American Elder Care, Sunshine State Health Plan, and United Healthcare. The MCO's by districts and county are set forth at http://www.floridalegal.org/medicaid.ltc./choosingamanagedplanformedicaidlongtermcare.

Current Medicaid recipients first receive a pre-welcome letter, then a welcome letter, and finally a reminder letter. These letters alert recipients to their upcoming deadline to choose a Plan and explain that if they fail to choose one they will be enrolled in a default Plan. The Agency for Health Care Administration will determine in which default plan the person will be enrolled. The determination is required to be based upon whether the plan's network of providers has the ability to meet the needs of the person, whether the person is already receiving services from one of the Plan's providers, and whether one plan has providers that are closer to the person's home than those of other plans.

Once a Medicaid recipient has chosen and enrolled in a Plan, that person will only have a limited amount of time before he or she is locked-in for the next twelve (12) months. After selecting a plan, individuals will only have a ninety day window in which to change. However, after the ninety day window has closed, the Florida Statutes only allow an individual to leave the Plan during the ensuing year if they can show "good cause." The Florida Statutes define good cause to include, but do not limit it to, poor quality of care, lack of access to necessary specialty services, unreasonable delay or denial of service, or fraudulent enrollment. Florida's Agency for Health Care Administration (AHCA) is required by this statute to make the determination as to whether good cause exists. However, the statute also states that AHCA may require an individual to use the Plan's grievance process before the agency will make this determination, unless there is immediate risk of permanent damage to the person's health. While Plans may give recipients the impression that they must bring their grievances through the Plan's internal appeal process, this is not legally accurate. If a Plan denies or reduces a recipient's benefits, the recipient has a right under Federal law to a Medicaid Fair Hearing. These hearings are conducted by the Florida Department of Children and Families. Medicaid recipients have the right under Federal law to a Fair Hearing when their benefits have been denied or reduced and should not be required to appeal through the Plan itself. A recipient may annually select a new plan within sixty days of the anniversary of the selection or placement in the plan. Recipients can contact a choice counselor online at www.flmedicaidmanagedcare.com or by telephone at (877) 711-3662.

Just Say No

It is possible in Florida for an institutionalized spouse to receive custodial nursing home assistance from the Department of Children and Families despite the community spouse having excess countable assets exceeding the community spouse resource allowance if the community spouse refuses to make the assets available for the institutionalized spouse's assistance. Florida's Economic Self-Sufficiency Public Assistance Policy Manual states in part:

If after declaring and verifying his assets, the community spouse refuses to make them available to the client, the institutionalized spouse may assign his rights of support to the state and obtain institutional care benefits, and the institutionalized spouse assigns to the State any rights to support from the community spouse by submitting the Assignment of Support Rights form referenced in a form signed by the institutionalized spouse or their representative.

Also, if the couple has been separated for a long time and the community spouse cannot be located, there is no "community spouse" and the applicant for Medicaid nursing home assistance must be considered an individual when applying income and asset standards.

Community spouses who refuse to make their assets available to the institutionalized spouse are not entitled to a community spouse income allowance.

The Department of Children and Families is automatically subrogated to any rights that a Medicaid applicant, recipient, or legal representative has to any third-party benefit for the full amount of medical assistance provided by Medicaid.

In Connor v. Southwest Florida Regional Medical Hospital, Inc., 668 So. 2d 175, (Fla. 1995), the Florida Supreme Court abrogated the common law doctrine of necessities between spouses. Thus, an action by the Florida Department of Children and Families against a community spouse for the Medicaid assistance provided the community spouse would likely be dismissed since a spouse in Florida has no duty to pay his or her spouse's creditors for necessaries.

Nevertheless, Florida Statute § 61.09 does state: "If a person having the ability to contribute to the maintenance of his or her spouse and support of his or her minor child fails to do so, the spouse who is not receiving support...may apply to the court for alimony without seeking dissolution..." While it is uncertain how the court will rule, the agent under a durable power of attorney for the institutionalized spouse may bring an action against the community spouse for the cost of the wife's care in the nursing home and then assign that support right to the Department of Children and Families.

CHAPTER 20

LONG-TERM CARE INSURANCE

- Long-Term Care Insurance
- Long-Term Care Insurance Partnership Program

Long-Term Care Insurance

Insurance coverage for long-term health care can reimburse a person for subsequent expenses related to a stay in a nursing home or assisted living facility or for home health care. Reimbursement for such services takes place when the beneficiary of the policy is unable to perform two or more activities of daily living or suffers from a cognitive impairment. The six activities of daily living are eating, toileting, transferring, bathing, dressing, and continence. A cognitive impairment is defined as a loss or deterioration in intellectual capacity that requires another person's substantial supervision or verbal cuing in order to perform activities of daily living.

The benefit level for a long-term care insurance policy should equal the average cost of long-term care services in the community where a person intends to reside if a need for long-term care services becomes necessary. It is important to know whether the policy will cover the full daily benefit for each day that services are needed or only the actual cost of the services. An annual increase in the daily benefit due to inflation should also be considered. The contract should indicate how many years it will pay for long-term care. Though three years is the normal term of coverage, a person may select a plan for a longer period, such as five years, six years, or a lifetime.

The elimination period represents the number of days that a person must reside in a long-term care facility before receiving benefits. The annual premium for the policy is normally less if the waiting period increases. Some policies do not require that this elimination period is longer. Some policies do not require that this waiting period consist of consecutive days.

A policy provision should require that the company notify a designated person (third party) when nonpayment threatens termination of the policy. That person is then given an additional period of time to pay the delinquent installments. This is important because of the possibility that the payments were not made because of a loss of mental ability on the part of the insured.

It is important that a person compare the provisions in several long-term policies before deciding on the best coverage for the premium he or she can afford. The coverage provided will vary based on the premium cost.

The Health Insurance Portability and Accessibility Act of 1996 clarified that eligible long-term care insurance premiums paid during a tax year for a qualified long-term care insurance contract can be included as an itemized deduction for medical expenses. However, the premium cannot exceed a specified dollar limit. It is important to remember that the amount of the medical expenses that can be deducted must exceed 10 percent of the taxpayer's adjusted gross income. However, the threshold will remain at 7 1/2 percent of adjusted gross income through the year 2016 if the taxpayer is age 65 or older. If a person does not itemize his or her deductions, there is no income tax benefit for paying long-term care insurance premiums. The limit on the amount of the premium for a qualified long-term care insurance contract that can be included as an itemized deduction for medical expenses is increased annually for the percentage by which the medical care component of the Consumer Price Index for August of the preceding year exceeds the component for August of the preceding year.

The maximum amount allowed for the annual medical expense deduction in the year 2015 for an individual who pays eligible long-term care premiums and has not attained age 41 at the end of the tax year is a dollar limit of $380 in 2015. A person between 41 and 50 at the end of this tax year can include up to $710 of the annual premium as an itemized medical expense in 2015. A person between the ages of 51 and 60 at the end of the tax year can include up to $1,430 of the annual premium as an itemized medical expense in 2015. An individual over 60 but not yet 71 at the end of the tax year can include an itemized medical expense up to $3,800 in 2015. An individual more than 70 years of age before the end of the tax year is limited in 2015 for premiums paid for a qualified long-term care insurance contract to $4,750 as a medical expense. A husband and a wife who are filing a joint income tax return may each include their annual premium paid at the appropriate limitation set forth above for a qualified long- term care insurance contract.

The Health Insurance Portability and Accessibility Act also clarified that the maximum amount of benefit excluded from income taxation pursuant to a qualified long-term care insurance contract was $330 per day in 2015. This amount is adjusted annually for inflation. A benefit payment in excess of this dollar limit is excluded from taxable income only to the extent that the individual has actually incurred additional costs for qualified long-term care services.

To avoid inclusion in income tax, the benefits received from a policy issued after January 1, 1997, must be from a qualified long-term care insurance contract. A qualified long-term care insurance contract provides that the insurance proceeds will be paid only for necessary diagnostic, preventative, therapeutic, curing, treating, mitigating, and rehabilitative services, and maintenance of personal care services. In addition, these services must be required by a chronically ill individual, and must follow a plan of care prescribed by a licensed health care practitioner. A chronically ill person is defined as an individual who has been certified by a licensed health care practitioner as being unable to perform, without substantial assistance from another, at least two out of the six daily living activities mentioned above for at least 90 days because the individual has lost the capacity to function. A contract is not considered a qualified long-term care insurance contract unless it takes into account at least five of the six activities in determining whether an individual is a chronically ill individual. A chronically ill person may also be a person who requires substantial supervision to protect him or her from injury because of his or her lack of awareness. The qualified policy must also offer the consumer the options of "inflation" and "nonforfeiture" protection, although the consumer can choose not to purchase these features.

A long-term care contract issued before 1997 that met the long-term care insurance requirements of that state and is intended to regulate its coverage is treated as a qualified long-term care insurance contract.

Long-Term Care Insurance Partnership Program

The Florida Legislature has approved Florida's participation in a federal program designed to encourage individuals to purchase long-term care insurance policies to cover future long-term care needs. A qualified long-term care insurance policy allows the Department of Children and Families to disregard special assets if the beneficiary of a qualified long-term care insurance policy applies for Medicaid nursing care. An individual who currently owns a long-term care policy should consider asking his or her insurance carrier to convert the present policy to the new qualified long-term care insurance partnership policy.

By example, if the long-term care insurance company pays out $60,000 for nursing home benefits for a beneficiary, the Department of Children and Families must subtract $60,000 from the individual's total countable assets when determining if the individual's total assets are within the Medicaid program limits. It is important that the long-term care insurance policy be certified under the standards established by the Office of Insurance Regulation as a qualified state LTC Insurance Partnership Policy.

CHAPTER 21

LIFE CARE PLANNING

Our modern health care systems are founded on the principles of acute care and are focused on curing the patient's immediate health care need or reacting to the pending health care crisis. However, there is another group of elderly clients who for many years have been neglected. These are the older clients who have chronic illness that require a continuity of care. Without assistance in the home or in assisted living facilities, these elderly clients will fall and break a hip, or perhaps injure themselves much more severely. This will of course result in skilled care and perhaps extended custodial care in a nursing home that could have been avoided with the implementation of a good home health care system.

Advanced age brings about functional impairments that will limit the elder's ability to perform one or more activities of daily living. The inability to perform these activities of daily living causes a person to depend on others for health care assistance to perform these necessary activities of daily living. In addition, cognitive impairments will also cause an elder to need supervision.

This year, about nine million men and women over the age of 65 will need a different form of long-term care assistance in the form of assistance with one or more activities of daily living. Twenty-five percent of these older adults are limited in their ability to perform activities of daily living. This number will increase to twelve million by 2020.

It is important to remember that an "impairment" does not mean that an institutionalized form of long-term care is required. It is only after a chronic condition takes its toll on the elder's health and self-care is no longer necessary that long-term care may become needed. When an elder experiences losses in the ability to function and assistance with activities of daily living become necessary, the elder must pick and choose from the many services that are available. The services that are selected must be specifically selected for that elder, and the extent of those services to be provided must also be determined. For instance, it means little to provide a person with cognitive dementia with physical rehabilitation. Instead, the person with dementia needs a sitter to provide supervision and a person who can dispense only the right medicines that may improve this person's cognitive functioning.

However, not all services selected for the elder may be affordable. For instance, assisted living for the most part is not paid for by Medicare or Medicaid. Often, a senior with early stage dementia is inappropriately placed in a nursing home because Medicaid pays for this form of custodial care and not assisted living. But, with "fine-tuning" the elder's home can be sold or a reverse mortgage taken. The elder can pay the difference between his or her social security and pension income and the cost of the assisted living facility with this additional lump sum for many years. In the alternative, VA Aid and Attendance may be available to defray the excess expense of assisted living over current income sources.

It is often thought that the government pays for no assistance to help someone who is incapacitated to remain in his or her home. But, if a person has an illness for which he or she needs medical care, as prescribed by his or her doctor and that person is homebound and the elder is a veteran or a widow of a veteran and has limited assets or income, there may be some home benefits available to the veteran or the veteran's spouse. In addition, many communities and charitable organizations have senior transportation services, homebound meal programs, adult day care programs, property tax relief, assistance with paying utility bills, homemaker assistance and sitter service. Many of these programs are coordinated by the local Area Agency on Aging. In addition, there are some Medicaid waiver programs.

Medicare does help an infirmed elder to some extent by providing skilled nursing facilities under the skilled nursing home coverage for at least 20 days, and an additional 80 days if the patient can afford the 20 day to 100 day deductible or has supplemental insurance. In addition, Medicaid will pay for custodial care in a nursing home for an indefinite period if the patient has not given away assets within the look-back period explained in Chapter 19 and countable assets below the eligibility limits.

A consideration may be to self insure for possible future care needs. Another source to pay for the immediate care needs is through the children's contributions and donated care. Of course, the sale of parcels of real property other than the homestead should be considered.

CHAPTER 22

ELDER MEDIATION AND SHARED FAMILY DECISION MAKING

Elder mediation assists an elderly person and family members or caregivers to resolve conflicts that naturally arise when this elderly person must make a transition that becomes necessary due to aging or to resolve other necessary issues affecting the elderly person's change in his or her status quo. This private mediation is an effective way for families and the elder to address and resolve these aging issues. The mediation is voluntary and the contents of the mediation are kept confidential by the mediator. The mediation empowers the older person to fully understand and agree to the solutions reached.

During the elder mediation the impartial third party known as the mediator assists the older persons, his or her family members, caregivers and others who are interested to have difficult conversations, make decisions and resolve conflicts that arise for the older adult as of these transitions. Elder mediation preserves the elder's independence while resolving the best caregiving needs, disability and estate planning needs of the elder. This process takes into consideration the community resources available to the elder, living arrangements, health care alternatives, Medicaid and other public assistance benefits. Support persons and advocates who are invited to the mediation may also participate in the conversations that occur during the mediation. All participants have the opportunity to speak and to be heard and to work together during the mediation to resolve the issues.

An Elder mediator recognizes the need for the senior to make appropriate choices while taking into consideration the physical, cognitive or social limitations of the senior while providing the maximum participation by the senior and the other parties in order to promote the senior's informed self-determination.

Similarly, a Shared Family Decision Making Agreement assists the elder's family members to work through their divergent opinions regarding who should care for the aging elder and the level care the elder should receive from each sibling. Without a family caregiver agreement between the children the vast majority of families fall back on one primary caregiver-often the daughter or child who lives closest to the parent. A Shared Family Decision Making Agreement permits the work assignments related to caring for the elder to be divided according to each child's available time and talents. One child may assume the responsibility of providing the care and attention for the elder or to look in on the parent who is placed in an assisted living facility with the pledged financial assistance of all of the children according to their financial abilities. Another child may assume the responsibility for managing the parent's assets, attending to the payment of the parent's bills and applying for reimbursement from insurance companies. An agreement should also be reached as to who will be the spokesperson for the parent in the event greater medical or custodial assistance becomes necessary. After dividing the tasks, the children might agree to have a designated time each week for a conference call to confirm that there is not a matter regarding the parent's care that is going unattended.

The Elder Mediator can facilitate an Elder Mediation or a Mediation that results in a Shared Family Decision Making Agreement between the siblings or other caregivers. Such an agreement often results in the avoidance of a costly and sometimes unnecessary guardianship proceeding.

CHAPTER 23

VIATICAL AND LIFE SETTLEMENT AGREEMENTS

The term viatical is derived from the Latin word viaticum, which means a supply of money or other necessities for a journey. In a viatical settlement, a person or a privately owned company agrees to purchase a life insurance policy or an interest in the life insurance policy from a person who has a catastrophic or life-threatening illness or condition. In exchange, the owner of the policy receives a percentage of the policy's face value, depending on his or her projected life expectancy, the projected cost of the remaining premiums due before death, and the time value of money.

The buyer of the policy will receive the full amount of the life insurance proceeds on the death of the insured. The proposed buyer of the life insurance policy is responsible for hiring a medical expert to review and evaluate the medical records to verify the terminal illness and to predict the insured's life expectancy. The buyer will also want to obtain the signed consents and releases from the insured's previously named policy beneficiary and from the insured's heirs. An attorney must then draft the assignment forms for the insured's signature. The discounted price for the policy being purchased is released to the insured as soon as the insurance company accepts the assignment of the policy to the buyer. A life settlement agreement works the same way and has no separate statute.

The Florida laws state that the Department of Insurance is not authorized to regulate the amount paid to the terminally ill patient for a policy. However, a viatical settlement provider is required to obtain a license from the Department of Insurance after a thorough background check of the principals of the company, as well as their ability to lawfully and successfully perform as a viatical settlement provider. Before obtaining a license, a viatical settlement provider must first deposit securities having a value of at least $100,000 in trust with the Florida Department of Insurance Commissioner, or deposit $25,000 in securities and post a surety bond acceptable to the department in the amount of $75,000. In addition, all applications, viatical settlement contract forms rating manuals, and other related forms proposed to be used by the viatical settlement provider must be approved by the Department of Insurance before a license will be issued.

The viatical settlement broker, or provider in transactions in which no broker is used, must first inform the policyholder prior to the date he or she applies for a viatical settlement contract that there are possible alternatives to viatical settlement contracts for persons having catastrophic or life-threatening illness, including but not limited to accelerated death benefits that may be offered by the insurer of the life insurance policy. The policyholder must also be informed that the proceeds of the viatical settlement could be taxable and that a tax advisor should first be consulted. The policyholder must be informed that the viatical settlement proceeds could be subject to creditor claims and that receiving these proceeds could adversely affect the recipient's eligibility for Medicaid or other government benefits or entitlement. Seeking advice from the appropriate agency is advised.

The policyholder must be informed that all viatical settlement contracts entered into in Florida must contain an unconditional rescission provision that allows the policyholder to rescind the contract within 15 days after the settlement proceeds are received. It is understood that, should this occur, the proceeds are returned. The policyholder must be informed of the name, business address, and telephone number of the escrow agent, and the fact that the policyholder may inspect or receive copies of all relevant escrow or trust agreements or documents. Before a viatical settlement provider enters an agreement, it must be ascertained whether the policyholder has any dependent children. If the policyholder has dependent children, he or she may not sell more than 50 percent of the face value of the policy.

The law states that a viatical settlement provider may not negotiate or enter into a contract to purchase a policy from a terminally ill patient if the policy contains an accelerated death benefit provision allowing benefits for a period that is equal to or exceeds the time period available under the viatical settlement contract, unless the issuer of the policy submits a written denial or refusal to provide such accelerated benefits.

A violation of this law is considered an unfair trade practice, and may also result in civil damages together with court costs and reasonable attorney fees incurred by the person bringing the action. If the court determines that the action was frivolous or harassing, the person bringing the action may be liable for the defendant's court costs and reasonable attorney fees.

CHAPTER 24

GRANDPARENT VISITATION

In 1984, the Florida Legislature passed a statute authorizing our courts to grant visitation rights to grandparents under certain limited circumstances. This court-ordered grandparent visitation was authorized for when the marriage of the parents of the child has been dissolved, a parent of the child has deserted the child, or the child was born out of wedlock and not later determined to be a child born within wedlock.

This statute required the court to first determine that such visitation would be in the best interest of the grandchild. In determining if this visitation was in the best interest of the grandchild, the Florida statute stated that the court was to consider the grandparent's willingness to encourage a close parent-child relationship, the length and quality of the prior grandparent-child relationship, the child's preference, the child's mental and physical health, and the grandparent's mental and physical health.

While never finding this statute to be completely unconstitutional, the Florida Supreme Court has systematically ruled that various provisions of this grandparent visitation statute are unenforceable. This court has repeatedly held that the state should not permit grandparents to interfere with parental rights to custody and control of children except in cases where the health and welfare of a child is threatened. Even assuming that grandparent visitation promotes the health and welfare of the child, our courts have consistently held that the state may only impose a grandparent visitation over the parent's objections on a showing that failing to do so would be harmful to the child. This right of a parent to be free from this form of governmental interference is based on protections afforded in the Fourteenth Amendment of the United States Constitution and the right of privacy provisions found in Article 1, Section 23 of our Florida Constitution.

All fifty states have statutes that provide for grandparent visitation in some form. In the year 2000, the United States Supreme Court confirmed in the case of Troxel v. Granville, 500 US 53 (US Sup. ct. 2000) that the Fourteenth Amendment to the United States Constitution permits a state to interfere with a parent's fundamental right to rear their children only when there is a showing of demonstrable harm to the child's health or welfare. Thus, only where there is a showing of substantial harm to the child by denying a grandparent visitation is the state's interest sufficiently compelling to warrant such governmental intrusion.

The harm to the grandchild often arises when a child loses a parent to illness or an accident and the surviving parent cuts off access to the deceased spouse's family. Often, the deceased spouse's parents have been a primary caretaker for the grandchild after school while the parents are still at work. In some cases, grandparent visitation is cut off when the spouse remarries. In these cases where the parents have allowed their child to closely bond with grandparents, a psychologist may find that the loss of that relationship can be equal to a child experiencing another death. This is especially true when a grandparent has been a regular caretaker and a psychological parent relationship has been formed between the child and grandparent.

Nevertheless, the legislature does recognize that many minor children in this state live with and are well cared for by members of their extended families. The parents of these children have often provided for their care by placing them temporarily with another family member who is better able to temporary care for them. However, such family members are unable to give complete care to the child in their custody because they lack a legal document that explains and defines their relationship to the child, and they are unable to effectively give consent to the care of the child by third parties. This includes consenting to necessary and reasonable medical and dental care and securing records necessary for the child's care including enrolling the child in school and doing other things necessary for the care of the child.

A petition for temporary or concurrent custody of a minor child can be filed with the court specifying the custody being requested, the services or actions the petitioner is unable to obtain or undertake. The court may then enter an order that it is in the best interest of the child for the petitioner to have temporary custody of the child and confirming the time the petitioner is allowed to have such temporary custody.

PART THREE
ESTATE PLANNING

CHAPTER 25

WILLS

The statement "Where there is a will, there is a way" might be said to apply equally well to a last will and testament. A valid will ensures that the assets a person worked a lifetime to acquire are distributed to beneficiaries the owner deems worthy.

If a person dies without a valid will or trust, or in other words intestate, a Florida statute dictates how the assets are distributed. This statute, which names certain heirs as beneficiaries, is inflexible and will apply regardless of the deceased person's desires or wishes. .A person must also recognize that circumstances change, and those changes will necessitate amending or revising the will. These changes are made in a codicil to a will.

A will is a document that directs the disposition of the person's property on or after his or her death. A will must be in writing and signed by the person making the will at the end, or the person making the will may direct that his or her name will be signed at the end by some other person in the presence of the person intending to make a will. The person signing the will or the person signing the will of another must also sign the will in the presence of at least two witnesses. These witnesses must sign the will in the presence of the person intending to make a will and in the presence of each other.

No particular form of words is necessary for a will to be valid if it is signed with the required formalities which are described in the previous paragraph.

A codicil is an amendment to a will. A codicil must also be signed with the same formalities as a will. A holographic will is a handwritten will that is not properly witnessed. A nuncupative will is an oral will declared or dictated by a person in his or her final sickness before a sufficient number of witnesses, and afterwards reduced to writing. The Florida statues do not authorize a judge to admit a holographic or a nuncupative will to probate. However, a will in a person's handwriting that has been signed and witnessed in the same manner for a will is not considered a holographic will and may be admitted to probate.

The purpose of probate is to collect a deceased person's assets, pay his or her claims, taxes, and administrative expenses from those assets, and distribute the remainder of the assets after administrative expenses to the beneficiaries entitled to receive them.

Any will, other than a holographic or nuncupative will, signed by a nonresident of Florida is valid as a will in Florida if it is valid under laws of the state or country where the will was signed. The problem with admitting such a will to probate is that unless the will is self-proved, a witness to the will in the state where it was signed must make an oath that the person who made the will was of sound mind and no undue influence when the will was signed. The probate of this will may be delayed while a commissioner (notary public) in the state where the person is making the will resided is appointed by a Florida circuit judge.

A valid will from another state or from Florida may be made self-proving when it is signed or at any subsequent date through the acknowledgment of the will by the person signing the will and the oaths of the witnesses which are made before an officer authorized to administer oaths such as a notary public. A self-proved will may be admitted to probate without the subsequent testimony of a witness to the will.

A will or a codicil, or any part of either, may be revoked by a subsequent will, codicil or other document declaring the revocation of the previous document, if the same formalities required for the execution of a will are observed in the execution of the new will, codicil or other writing. The revocation of a subsequent will which revoked a previous will does not revive the previous will, even though the previous will is in existence at the date of the revocation of the subsequent will. A will or codicil may also be revoked by the person making the will, or some other person in the presence of the person who made the will and at his or her direction, by burning, tearing, canceling, defacing, obliterating, or destroying it with the intention, and for the purpose of, revocation. There cannot be a partial revocation of a will by these actions. Thus, a person cannot vary the terms of his or her will after it's signing by alterations or changes of its face that gives new meaning to the part altered, unless the alterations or changes are signed and attested to in the manner provided by law for the making of a will.

It is important to remember that the person named as the personal representative (executor) may not be qualified to serve in Florida. For instance, if that person does not reside in Florida or is not a relative or a spouse of a relative, he or she cannot serve as the personal representative.

While spouses can contract to not make a new will after the death of the first spouse, it is important to remember that a contract not to revoke a will does not prohibit the surviving spouse from giving away these assets before he or she dies. However, the surviving spouse will then be deprived of the assets during his or her remaining lifetime.

Under Florida law, if no will is signed by a spouse before his or her death, the surviving spouse will receive all of the deceased spouse's estate if there are no lineal descendants of the deceased or all of the lineal descendants are the lineal descendants of the surviving spouse. If there are lineal descendants of the deceased who are not lineal descendants of the surviving spouse, the surviving spouse will receive one-half of the probate estate.

It is important to remember that a new will should be signed after the marriage or a will signed before the marriage should specifically provide for the new spouse or specifically disinherit the new spouse.

A surviving spouse is also entitled to a life estate in the decedent's homestead or elect joint ownership within six months and to receive an allowance for his or her living expenses during the administration of the estate of the deceased spouse. This allowance was recently increased by the Florida legislature to a maximum of $18,000. The amount of the allowance is determined by the circuit judge. A surviving spouse is also entitled to elect to receive the deceased's household furnishings having a net value of $20,000 as of the date of death and two motor vehicles held in the decedent's name and regularly used by the decedent or members of the decedent's immediate family as their personal vehicles. However, the gross vehicle weight of each vehicle cannot have a weight in excess of 15,000 pounds. This election must be filed with the clerk of the court where the probate is being administered within 4 months after the date of service of the notice of administration on the surviving spouse.

A surviving spouse may waive wholly or partly his or her rights to share in the probate estate, to receive exempt property, to take a family allowance and to receive the use of the homestead. This waiver can be executed before or after marriage by a written contract, and it must be signed by the party waiving any right. Each spouse must make a fair disclosure to the other spouse of his or her assets if the agreement or waiver is executed after marriage. No disclosure is required for an agreement or waiver before marriage.

CHAPTER 26

TRUSTS

- Revocable Trust

- Irrevocable Trust

- Florida's Trust Code

A trust established during the lifetime of the person creating the trust is a living trust. In contrast, a trust created at death in a last will and testament is a testamentary trust.

A settlor or grantor is a person creating the trust. When a living trust is established, a trustee must be appointed to manage and later distribute the trust assets to the beneficiaries. The beneficiaries are the persons who ultimately receive the assets from the trust. This event normally occurs upon the death of the settlor or grantor. The living trust instructs the trustee how to manage the assets and when to distribute the assets to the beneficiaries named in the trust. The person creating the trust can also be a beneficiary of the trust during his or her lifetime.

The person creating the trust (the settlor or grantor) may serve as the trustee of the trust. In such event, a successor trustee is named in the trust to manage and distribute the trust assets if the settlor or grantor is subsequently incapable of serving as trustee as a result of his or her disability or death.

Only assets conveyed to the trust can be administered by the trustee who owns the legal title to the trust assets for the benefit of the beneficiaries. The person creating the trust must convey real property to the trust by a properly executed deed. Likewise, personal property must be transferred to the trustee by a properly executed bill of sale. Bank accounts, stock certificates, certificates of deposits, and other intangible assets must be retitled in the name of the trustee.

Assets not conveyed or transferred to the trustee are subject to probate. A pour-over will is used to distribute to the trustee assets not owned by the trustee when the settlor or grantor dies. These assets are then administered and distributed to the beneficiaries named in the trust.

Revocable Trust

A trust established during the lifetime of the grantor or settlor is either revocable or irrevocable. A revocable trust permits the grantor or settlor to revoke the trust, alter the terms of the trust, or withdraw some or all of the assets from the trust. A revocable trust becomes irrevocable upon the death of the grantor or settlor.

Since the grantor or settlor of a living trust retains control of assets through his or her power to revoke or alter the trust, there are no gift, income, and estate tax consequences when assets are conveyed to a revocable trust. The grantor or settlor continues to report the earnings of the trust assets on his or her personal income tax return if the grantor or settlor is the trustee.

The constitution of the state of Florida and the Florida statutes grant a homestead exemption to every person who has legal or equitable title to real estate and maintains a permanent residence on that property for himself or herself and family. If this residence is placed in a revocable trust, the owner may still claim the homestead tax exemption as long as he or she is the sole beneficiary of the trust during his or her lifetime. The owner must also be permanently residing on the real property owned by the trust. In the trust, the grantor must be granted the sole right to the full use, occupancy, and possession of this homestead. Also, the revocable trust must not grant the trustee any power, authority, or duty with respect to the homestead until the person creating the trust directs otherwise or revokes the trust agreement, or the beneficiary dies.

The living trust is an excellent instrument by which a person can plan for the administration of assets in the event of a disability. A successor trustee can be named to administer the trust assets in such an event. The trust instrument normally states that when the written opinions of licensed physicians (the grantors and another physician) certify that the grantor is physically or mentally incapable of managing his or her property, the grantor's right to continue to serve as the trustee during that period of incapacity is suspended. The trust document normally reserves the right of the person creating the trust to request the court to determine the question of incapacity or capacity to manage the trust assets. The successor trustee will manage the trust assets during the period of the trustee's incapacity.

The need for a living trust is based on many factors, including the amount of the assets, the ability of the spouse to continue to manage assets acquired during the marriage, and the health of the husband and wife. Though it is best to consider a living trust as soon as the circumstances justify, the need for a living trust should especially be evaluated upon the death of the spouse. Special consideration should be given to the availability of a child to serve as successor trustee. If the child is not available to serve as the successor trustee, serious consideration should be given to the appointment of a bank or trust company as the successor, or perhaps the initial trustee.

The assets placed in a living trust are not subject to a probate proceeding. However, these assets must be administered after the death of the settlor or grantor. The successor trustee must collect the trust assets, pay the final bills, be responsible for the federal estate tax apportioned to the trust, and make distribution of the remaining assets according to the trust's instructions. Creditors in a probate proceeding must file claims against probate assets within three months of the first publication of a notice to creditors in the newspaper. Since there is no similar publication procedure to shorten the claim period for a trust, a successor trustee cannot distribute the trust assets to beneficiaries free of potential creditor claims for two years from the date of the grantor's death. This is because the statute of limitations period within which creditor claims must be asserted extends for two years from the date of the grantor's or settlor's death. A summary probate administration can be useful, since this procedure permits publication of a notice requiring that creditors file claims within three months of the date of first publication. If a claim is not filed in the summary probate administration within three months of the date of first publication, the claim is barred. A summary administration can be used to probate the deceased's tangible personal property such as furniture. The assets used for the summary administration cannot have a fair market value exceeding $75,000.

Irrevocable Trust

Another form of trust is an irrevocable trust. This is a trust that cannot be amended or altered. The assets conveyed to an irrevocable trust cannot be withdrawn or returned to the grantor or settlor. An irrevocable trust is normally created for estate tax purposes. A person will transfer assets to an irrevocable trust to avoid having to include the fair market value of these assets in his or her taxable estate at death. It is important to remember that a transfer of an asset to an irrevocable trust constitutes a gift. Accordingly, the fair market value of the asset on the date of the transfer to the trust must be reported to the Internal Revenue Service as a gift by April 15 after the year of the transfer. The taxpayer's estate or gift tax unified credit will be applied to the gift taxes due as a result of this transfer. The advantage of transferring assets to an irrevocable trust is that the appreciation in the value of these assets will not be subject to federal estate taxes upon the taxpayer's death.

Another use of the irrevocable trust is for the purchase of life insurance to provide the beneficiaries of the trust with the money to pay the estate taxes of the grantor or settlor. Since the life insurance policy is owned by the trustee and not the taxpayer, the proceeds paid on the taxpayer's death are not included in his or her gross estate. The payment of the premium for the life insurance during the taxpayer's life is normally made from annual contributions by the taxpayer to the trustee of the irrevocable trust. Since there is presently a $14,000 per donee annual exclusion for federal gift tax purposes, there is no gift tax owed when these annual contributions to the irrevocable trust are made if the beneficiaries of the trust are granted the unrestricted right to withdraw these contributions during the year in which they are paid to the trustee. The withdrawal right for each beneficiary is usually limited to the amount of the annual gift tax exclusion, which is presently $14,000 per donee.

The proceeds of an existing life insurance policy transferred to an irrevocable trust will be included in the estate of the grantor or settlor if he or she fails to survive for three years after the date of the transfer. Also, there is a gift tax on the value of the life insurance policy on the date of the transfer to the irrevocable trust.

If avoiding probate on the distribution of an asset after death is a goal, there are methods other than a trust. Bank accounts can be distributed to others without a living trust or a probate proceeding through the creation of joint bank accounts with the right of survivorship. However, there is the possibility of a withdrawal of funds by a joint owner without the knowledge and consent of the owner of the account.

Florida's Trust Code

Florida's new trust code became effective on July 1, 2007. With a few exceptions, the new statutes apply to all trusts whether created before or after July 1, 2007. This new trust code was necessary because Florida's trust law that existed prior to July 1, 2007 covered only a portion of the issues that arise in the administration of trusts. Many laws applicable to trusts and the rights of creditors to trust assets were found in other statutes or not at all. This new Trust code permits the person establishing a trust to appoint or designate a person to represent and bind a trust beneficiary or to receive notices, information, reports and accounts on the beneficiary's behalf. This is important if the person establishing the trust believes that the beneficiary may not be reasonably available or responsible to sign receipts and to communicate with the trustee. Thus, an attorney or a family member could accept notices and information and bind the beneficiary who may not communicate. This will save considerable expense related to unnecessary court hearings to approve accountings or to obtain necessary approvals needed by the trustee.

The person receiving a notice as a designated representative is not a fiduciary. He or she is not liable for acts or omissions made in good faith. The trustee cannot serve as designated representative. Another beneficiary may only serve as a representative if the beneficiary to be designated is a spouse, grandparent, or descendant of a grandparent of either the beneficiary being represented or that beneficiary's spouse. An amendment to an existing trust can be drafted by the attorney and signed by the person who has already created a trust to designate the appointment of a designated representative.

The new Florida Trust Code confirms that a trust is valid in Florida if it complies with either the law of the place where executed or the law where the person establishing the trust is domiciled at the time of creation. However, a trust for owning real property in Florida must comply with our Florida statutes requiring that a trust for land must be in writing and signed before witnesses by the party authorized to create the trust for the land. The new trust code confirms that the testamentary aspects of a revocable trust signed by a person who is domiciled in Florida at the time of execution are invalid unless the trust instrument is signed with the formalities required for the execution of a will in this state. The new trust code confirms that the capacity to create a trust is the same needed for the execution of a will. This new law confirms that a trust or portion thereof may be void if the creation of the trust is procured by fraud, duress, mistake, or undue influence. The new trust code clarifies that a trust must name a definite beneficiary or a charity and confirms that a trust can be established for the care of an animal alive during the settlor's lifetime. The new laws permit a trust to be established for a charitable purpose for no longer than 21 years if the trustee is directed to apply the income annually to such worthy purposes as the trustee selects. A new provision in the Florida trust code permits the non-judicial modification of a trust after the grantor's or settlor's death. Thus, the trust can be modified by the unanimous agreement of the trustee and the living persons who are current, intermediate, and first remainder beneficiaries. However, the new law states that there cannot be a non-judicial modification if there is a provision in the trust that prohibits its amendment or revocation. It is accordingly important that a person consider amending his or her trust if no non-judicial amendment is to be permitted after death. The new law again provides that a trust consisting of property under $50,000 may be terminated if the trustee concludes the value of the trust property is insufficient to justify the cost of administration. However, the person creating the trust can expressly provide that the trust may be terminated even in this event.

This new trust code states that if a revocable trust is created or funded by more than one person, each person creating the trust may revoke or amend the trust with regard to the portion of the trust property attributable to that person's contribution. If there is a revocation or amendment of the trust by fewer than all the person's creating the trust, the trustee shall promptly notify the other persons creating the trust of the revocation or amendment. A new provision in the trust code states that an action contesting the validity of the revocable trust that was revocable at the time the person creating the trust died is barred, if not commenced within the earlier of the time as provided in the Florida statute of limitations or six months after the trustee has sent a person a copy of the trust instrument and a notice informing the person of the trust's existence, the trustees name and address, and of the time allowed for commencing a proceeding. A person who has created a revocable trust should consider setting an appointment with his or her attorney to review these and other changes in Florida's new trust code. A decision can then be made regarding the need to amend the existing trust to take advantage of these new laws.

CHAPTER 27

PRENUPTIAL AGREEMENTS

Anyone considering a second marriage should also consider signing a prenuptial agreement with his or her intended spouse. The purpose of this agreement is to promote each individual's mutual welfare and happiness in the marriage and to avoid disharmony, misunderstanding, and uncertainty during the marriage, or after the marriage ends due to divorce or death.

The intention of such an agreement is for both parties to define and limit the rights and interests concerning the property they have acquired prior to the marriage that they are about to enter. The agreement gives them separate rights to dispose of the property they owned during their lifetimes and at their deaths. It defines the rights and obligations of each person regarding the property each owns separately at the time of marriage, and any property acquired while in the new marriage, and specifies what will happen to that property should the couple separate or divorce.

A prenuptial agreement is signed by the parties prior to the marriage, in order to avoid the need for a judge to decide how the couple's assets will be distributed in the event of a divorce. Often, individuals contemplating a second marriage come to that union with children from the first marriage and an accumulation of assets from the previous marriage. The rights and obligations will differ from those of the first marriage when the parties were younger.

A prenuptial agreement should disclose and include a waiver of a subsequent claim to any of the other parties' assets and especially the following assets:

1. all financial information: a list of bank accounts, certificates of deposit, cash equivalents,
2. bonds and securities
3. partnerships
4. retirement benefits or accounts
5. IRA accounts
6. insurance and annuity contracts
7. motor vehicles
8. jewelry, collections, and antiques
9. miscellaneous personal property
10. notes, receivable, or other claims
11. indebtedness such as property taxes owed, credit card balances, mortgages, and claims.

Since the cost of medical and long-term nursing care for an older person can be considerable, it is important to confirm that sufficient funds have been reserved to pay for the medical and nursing expenses that will not be paid by Medicare. Alternatively, it should be confirmed that each party has (and intends to keep in force during the marriage) a supplemental health insurance policy as well as a long-term nursing care policy.

It is also important to remember that a spouse will have the authority to make medical decisions for the other spouse who is not capable of making health care decisions unless a health care surrogate has previously been designated. Therefore, spouses should sign health care advance directives and pre-need guardian statements that confirm the person they want to make their medical decisions and manage their assets in the event of a disability.

Prior to the second marriage, consideration should be given to whether any retirement benefits being received as a result of the death of a first spouse will terminate in the event of remarriage.

A divorce in a marriage in which the health of one spouse has declined can result in the other spouse being responsible for continuing support of that spouse through temporary alimony, permanent alimony, or rehabilitative alimony even after the second marriage has ended. The parties can sign a prenuptial agreement prior to the marriage in which they waive any claim for support in the event of a divorce. A prenuptial agreement is also necessary for each party to waive the right to receive a portion of the other's estate in the event of death. Without a prenuptial agreement, the new spouse is entitled to claim at least the elective share, which is 30 percent of the value of the deceased's elective estate. For further information, please refer to the chapter entitled Florida's New Elective Estate. The surviving spouse is also entitled to a life estate in the deceased spouse's homestead or joint property, a family allowance set by the circuit judge not to exceed $18,000, and household furniture having a net value of not more than $20,000, and two motor vehicles held in the decedent's name and regularly used by the decedent or members of the decedent's immediate family as their personal vehicles. However, the gross vehicle weight of each vehicle cannot have a weight in excess of 15,000 pounds.

A postnuptial agreement can be signed by spouses after the marriage to waive some or all marital rights. The parties should seek the advice of separate attorneys before signing a prenuptial or postnuptial agreement.

CHAPTER 28

FLORIDA'S ELECTIVE ESTATE

Until October 1, 2001, the surviving spouse of a person who died while having his or her permanent residence in Florida had the right to elect to receive only a share of the deceased spouse's probate estate. This elective share was equal to 30 percent of all property of the deceased spouse wherever located that is subject to probate administration except for real property not located in Florida.

This statute had been the subject of concern for several years. This is because many assets are often owned in a trust or a survivorship account and are not subject to probate administration. The spouse's elective share did not apply to these assets which are not subject to probate. In addition, there was no right under Florida law to claim an elective share in a second home owned by the deceased spouse in another state.

The need for the surviving spouse's share to encompass both probate and non-probate assets had been obvious for several years. The Florida legislature finally approved legislation regarding this subject that applies to all permanent residents of Florida. This statute that became effective on October 1, 2001, states that a spouse of a person who dies a permanent resident of Florida will have the right to elect to receive 30 percent of the deceased spouse's elective estate. The elective estate includes an interest in the following assets:

1. The decedent's Florida probate estate and real property the decedent owned in another state.
2. The decedent's interest in accounts or securities registered in Pay on Death, Transfer on Death, In trust for, or co-ownership with right of survivorship form.
3. The decedent's interest in property held in joint tenancy with right of survivorship or in tenancy by the entirety (husband and wife). In the case of accounts held in tenancy by the entirety, one-half the value of the account or security will be considered the interest of the deceased.
4. The decedent's property which is owned by his or her revocable trust. One half of the value of trust property will be included in the determination of the elective estate if the surviving spouse is the other owner of the revocable trust.
5. The decedent's beneficial interest in the net cash surrender value immediately before the death of any policy of life insurance on the decedent's life.
6. The value of amounts payable to or for the benefit of any person by reason of surviving the decedent under any public or private pension, retirement, or deferred compensation plan.

7. Property transferred during the one-year period preceding the death of the spouse.

There is exclusion for any transfer of property for medical or educational expenses and the first $14,000 of property transferred which qualifies for annual exclusion from U.S. gift taxes.

The statute permits the estate of the deceased spouse to satisfy the surviving spouse's share of the elective estate with the proceeds from a term or other form of insurance policy on the decedent's life. This statute also permits the spouse to establish an elective share trust wherein the surviving spouse has right to income for life payable at least as often as annually. During the remainder of the surviving spouse's life, no person other than the spouse can have the right to receive a distribution of income or principal to anyone other than the surviving spouse. The spouse's interest in the trust will be valued at a minimum of 50 percent of the underlying value of the trust property if the surviving spouse is to only receive the net income. That percentage will rise to 80 percent if the spouse or the trustee has the right to invade trust principal for the spouse's health, support, and maintenance. The percentage is increased to 100 percent if the spouse has the right to a general power of appointment.

With the extension of the elective estate to now include the deceased spouse's revocable trust, a standard revocable trust established before the death of the first spouse will no longer exclude these assets from being considered available to the surviving spouse for Medicaid purposes. However, the new statute authorizes the creation of a qualifying special needs trust in which the trustee has the discretion to pay the income and principal to only the surviving spouse during the remainder of his or her life. This statute states that if the trust is approved by the circuit judge, the elective share right of a surviving spouse will not extend to property held in this form of trust for an ill or disabled spouse. However, property passing to such a trust qualifies dollar for dollar in satisfaction of the spouse's elective share right.

The value of the property considered for the elective estate is the fair market value of the property on the date of the decedent's death, computed after deducting all claims, paid or payable from the elective estate and all mortgages, liens, or security interests on the property. The statute requires the surviving spouse to make the election within the earlier of six months from the date of service of the Notice of Administration on the surviving spouse or two years after the date of the decedent's death.

CHAPTER 29

FEDERAL ESTATE AND GIFT TAX LAW

- Federal Estate and Gift Tax Laws

- Federal Estate Tax Return

- No Florida Estate Tax

- Determining the Gross Estate

- Basis in Property Received From a Decedent Who Dies in 2015

- Basis in Property Received During His or Her Lifetime

- Portability of Unused Exemption Between Spouses

- Gift Tax Annual Exclusion

Federal Estate and Gift Tax Laws

There is a federal gift tax imposed on lifetime transfers of property and a federal estate tax is imposed on transfers of property at death. An exception is made when the lifetime or death transfer is made to a qualified charity. There is another transfer tax that is imposed when a substantial gift or devise is made to a person in a generation that is more than one generation younger than the person making the transfer. This is known as the generation transfer tax.

The American Taxpayer Relief Act was passed by Congress on January 2, 2013. It provides for a permanent continuation of the $5,000,000 exclusion from the estate, gift and generation-skipping tax and the continued unification for the exclusion of the estate, gift and generation-skipping tax purposes. This exemption is adjusted annually for inflation. The exclusion increased to $5,430,000 for 2015.This inflation adjustment is based on the one-year movement in the Consumer Price Index – All Urban Customers (CPI-U), as measured after August of each year. The maximum tax of 40% will apply to all gifts, devises and generation skipping transfers that are made by an individual in 2015 in excess of $5,430,000. It is important to understand that the $5,430,000 million exclusion is cumulative. Thus, a gift of $3,000,000, in 2012 will mean that only $2,430,000, is available in 2015 to gift without the payment of a federal gift tax. Likewise, a person who has made gifts during his or her lifetime of $5,430,000 will have no subsequent gift or estate tax exclusion in the year 2015, with the exception of the $14,000 annual gift tax exclusion explained below.

Federal Estate Tax Return

If a person has at the time of death an estate that does not exceed a gross value of $5,340,000, then there is no federal estate tax and this person's personal representative will not be required to file with the Internal Revenue Service a Federal Estate Tax return form 706. However, this return may still be filed for other reasons, such as locking in the date of death values of the decedent's assets to establish their stepped up basis explained below or to allocate the decedent's unused generation skipping transfer tax exemption to testamentary trusts created under the decedent's estate plan.

If it is determined that a person does have an estate with a gross value of more than $5,430,000 then this completed Federal Estate Tax Return form 706 must be filed with the Internal Revenue Service within 9 months after the date of the decedent's death. It is possible to file for an automatic 6 month's extension of this deadline. However, the application for the extension must be filed before the 9 month due date.

No Florida Estate Tax

Prior to 2005, the State of Florida had a state estate tax that was a percentage of the federal estate tax but was collected by the Florida Department of Revenue. This was called the "pick up tax." The "pick up tax" was phased out by Congress in 2005. The American Taxpayer Relief Act did not revive the pick up tax. Thus, Florida has no separate estate tax.

Determining the Gross Estate

To know whether a deceased person's estate will be liable for federal estate taxes in 2015, the person's gross estate first needs to be determined. A gross estate (for federal estate tax purposes) includes all property that the deceased owned or had an interest in at his or her death. The gross estate of a deceased person also includes the fair market value of property owned jointly with another except to the extent the other owner contributed toward the purchase of the property. However, for a husband and wife, there is a special 50-percent ownership rule for their jointly owned property, generally causing it to be treated as being owned equally by each spouse, regardless of who originally paid the purchase price.

The gross estate for federal estate tax purposes is comprised of the fair market value on the date of death of all stocks, bonds, tangible personal property, real property, cash, promissory notes, and the proceeds of life insurance policies owned by the deceased at death or under certain circumstances, within three years of his or her death.

The fair market value of the gross estate is determined as of the date of the individual's death or six months after death. The second value is known as the alternate valuation date that is allowed if the value of the gross estate is reduced and the election decreases the estate tax due the Internal Revenue Service.

Once the gross estate is determined, this amount is then reduced by funeral expenses, administration expenses, and debts and losses not reimbursed by insurance. Also, through the marital deduction, the taxable estate is reduced by whatever amount is left to the surviving spouse who is a United States citizen. The marital deduction can be taken for assets transferred to a marital deduction trust. The marital deduction trust must distribute to the surviving spouse all the net income earned on the trust assets at least annually and as much of the assets of the trust as are necessary for the surviving spouse's health, education, maintenance, and support. In the alternative, the marital deduction trust must assure to the surviving spouse all the net income earned on the trust assets at least annually and also grant the surviving spouse a general power of appointment to state who will receive the remaining trust principal upon his or her death. The assets allocated to the marital deduction will not be subject to federal estate taxes when the first spouse dies, but may be subject to estate tax at the death of the second spouse.

Basis in Property Received From a Decedent Who Dies in 2015

Property passing from a decedent who dies during 2015 takes a "stepped-up" basis. The basis of property passing to a beneficiary from a decedent's estate or revocable trust is the fair market value of the asset on the date of the decedent's death. In the alternative, the personal representative (executor) of the estate of the person making the transfer at death can elect an alternate valuation date that is the earlier of six months after the decedent's death or the date the property is sold or distributed by the estate. This step-up-in-basis generally eliminates the recognition of income on any appreciation of the property that occurred prior to the decedent's death. If the value of property on the date of the decedent's death is less than its adjusted basis, the property takes a "stepped-down" basis when it passes from a decedent's estate. The reason why the stepped up or stepped-down basis is important is that a person must pay a federal income tax on the amount realized from the sale of the property less the taxpayer's adjusted basis in this property.

Basis in Property Received During His or Her Lifetime

Basis generally represents a taxpayer's investment in property and the cost of capital improvements made to the property less any depreciation deductions taken with respect to the property before it is sold. When a person receives a gift of property during the lifetime of the person making the gift, the donee (person receiving the property) acquires the donor's basis. This is called the carryover basis. "Carryover basis" means that the basis in the hands of the donee is the same as it was in the hands of the donor. The basis of property transferred by lifetime gift also is increased, but not above fair market value, by any gift tax paid by the donor. The basis of a lifetime gift, however, generally cannot exceed the property's fair market value on the date of the gift. If the basis of property is greater than the fair market value of the property on the date of the gift, then, for purposes of determining loss, the basis is the property's fair market value on the date of the gift. The reason why the basis is important is that a person must pay a federal income tax on the amount realized from the sale of the property less the taxpayer's adjusted basis in this property.

Portability of Unused Exemption Between Spouses

Every U.S. citizen has an exclusion against federal estate and gift taxes. This exclusion avoids the payment of a federal estate and gift tax in 2015 on assets having a value of $5,430,000. This is called the applicable exclusion amount. For U.S. citizens dying after December 31, 2010, the amount of this exclusion that remains unused at by a deceased spouse can be applied by the surviving spouse to the estate or gift tax owed on assets subsequently transferred by the surviving spouse. The unused exclusion of deceased spouse is referred to as the Deceased Spouse's Unused Exclusion (DSUE). However, a deceased spouse's unused exclusion amount is only available to a surviving spouse if an election to preserve this unused exclusion is made on the deceased spouse's timely filed estate tax return, regardless of whether the estate of the predeceased spouse is otherwise required to file a federal estate tax return. This is called the portability election. It is important to remember that federal estate tax return must be filed within nine months of the date of death unless an extension is granted by the Internal Revenue Service.

It is accordingly important for a spouse to consider providing in his or her last will and testament that the Personal Representative (executor) shall make the portability election for any portion of the applicable exclusion amount that would otherwise be unused, even if it appears unclear that the surviving spouse or the surviving spouse's estate could benefit from such exclusion. It might be argued by the heirs of the deceased spouse that the expense related to the preparation of the federal estate tax return is unnecessary. Accordingly, a spouse should consider providing in his or her last will and testament that all expenses associated with making this election shall be an expense of the deceased spouse's administration.

It is important to remember that if the surviving spouse remarries and the new spouse predeceases the surviving spouse, the new spouse's DSUE amount replaces the DSUE amount of the first deceased spouse, and the benefit of the DSUE of the first spouse is lost. Thus, the surviving spouse's making gifts and using the DSUE amount as soon as possible after the death of the first spouse eliminates the possibility of losing this exclusion due to remarriage and removes all future appreciation in the assets given by the surviving spouse from his or her taxable estate. This saves estate taxes on the subsequent appreciation of these assets.

While it has always been considered best to establish a By-Pass Trust for the benefit of the surviving spouse, it is important to remember that assets transferred from the deceased spouse's estate to a credit shelter trust for the surviving spouse will not receive a stepped-up basis adjustment upon the death of the surviving spouse. Furthermore, while the assets remain in the By-Pass Trust, any undistributed taxable income above $11,950 of taxable income will be subject to the highest income tax rates at the trust level. Whereas, assets devised to a marital deduction QTIP will receive a stepped-up basis upon the death of the surviving spouse.

By example, if the first spouse has $5 million in assets when he or she dies, the traditional by-pass trust plan will result in splitting his or her taxable estate so that $2.5 million will be applied to the first spouse's credit shelter trust for the benefit of the surviving spouse and the first spouse retains his or her remaining assets in a marital deduction trust. Assume that the first spouse dies in 2015, and during the surviving spouse's subsequent lifetime all of the assets double in value, and that upon the surviving spouse's death the portability feature is still part of the law. There will be no federal estate taxes owed on the death of the second spouse if the portability election is timely made on the death of the first spouse since the surviving spouse will have a $7.5 million estate tax exclusion. In addition, the DSUE amount and the surviving spouse's applicable exclusion amount will grow with the cost-of-living index. However, the assets transferred to the credit shelter trust for the benefit of the surviving spouse will not receive a step up in basis at the surviving spouse's death. At a 23.8% rate of income taxation, the potential capital gain on the appreciation of the assets transferred to the credit shelter trust will be subject to a $595,000, capital gain income tax when the heirs of this credit shelter trust subsequently sell these assets after the death of the surviving spouse. In this example, if the husband and wife had owned all of their assets in joint names with right of survivorship or in tenancy by the entirety or all the assets were held in the husband's marital deduction QTIP trust, there would be no federal estate tax and no potential capital gain tax to the heirs of these assets. This is because all of these assets will receive a step up in basis upon the death of the surviving spouse.

However, it should be remembered that the non-federal estate tax advantages for continuing to use a By-Pass Trust plan on the death of the first spouse include asset management by a professional trustee, asset protection pursuant to spendthrift trust protection, and disposition control by the decedent spouse thus preventing the surviving spouse from diverting the assets to non-family members after the death of the first spouse.

Gift Tax Annual Exclusion

Donors of lifetime gifts are allowed an annual exclusion from a gift tax in 2015 of up to $14,000 on transfers of present interests in property to each donee during a taxable year. If the non-donor spouse consents to split the gift with the donor spouse, then the annual exclusion can be up to $28,000 per donee for 2015.

Chapter 30

CHARITABLE GIVING

- Deductions for Present Contributions
- Deferred Giving
- Charitable Remainder Trust
- Charitable Lead Trust
- Gift Annuities
- Pooled Income Fund

Deductions for Present Contributions

For federal income tax purposes, a taxpayer can deduct cash contributions to publicly supported charitable organizations, hospitals, churches, schools, and universities up to 50 percent of his or her adjusted gross income. A taxpayer who donates securities or real estate owned for more than a year to these organizations can deduct the fair market value of the property up to 30 percent of his or her adjusted gross income. Fair market value is defined as the price that property would sell for between a willing buyer and a willing seller, with neither being required to buy or sell and both having reasonable knowledge of the relevant facts.

A person may choose to increase his or her income tax deduction for long-term held securities or real estate to 50 percent of adjusted gross income by electing to deduct the gift on the basis of what it cost to purchase the securities, or cost basis, rather than its fair market value.

A person who donates real estate or securities owned for less than one year is limited to a deduction equal to the adjusted cost basis and not the fair market value of the gift. However, a person can deduct the value of this gift up to 50 percent of his or her adjusted gross income.

If a gift of cash is made to a private foundation, the charitable deduction is limited to 30 percent of the donor's contribution base, again with a five-year carry forward. Excess contributions not deducted the same year in which the gifts are made generally can be carried over and deducted over the next five years. However, this carryover expires with the death of the donor. If a donor who wants to make gifts in excess of this year's contribution limit is in frail health and married to a healthy spouse, the donor should consider transferring the property to be contributed to the healthy spouse. Then the healthy spouse can make the gift and continue to receive the benefit of the carryover in subsequent years after the death of the spouse in frail health.

The deductible limit for charitable contributions made by corporations is 10 percent of taxable income. The amount of any corporate gift in excess of the 10 percent limit may be carried forward and deducted until exhausted in the five years following the year of the gift. Charitable contributions made by S corporations flow through to the individual returns of the shareholders. The shareholder's deduction for contributions made by the corporation is limited to his or her basis in the S corporations stock, and any deduction will reduce the basis of that stock.

There are no percentage limits on the estate and gift tax deductions for charitable gifts. A canceled check alone is not considered sufficient evidence of a gift to a charity if the contribution is for more than $250. The taxpayer must have received a written acknowledgment of the gift from the charity. Such a letter or receipt must be received before the taxpayer/contributor claims the donation as a deduction on the tax return or it will be lost, even if it otherwise was legitimately deductible.

This letter or receipt of a gift needs to describe the amount of the cash contribution, a description of the property contributed and a description and good faith estimate of any goods or services provided to the contributor in return for the donation. Separate contributions of less than $250 to a single charity generally are not combined as a $250 contribution. For example, weekly contributions to a church usually are not totaled to meet the $250 limit. This exception, though, does not apply when multiple checks are written to the same charity on the same day.

A charity that receives a contribution of more than $75 with the intention of returning to the contributor something of value, such as a fine dinner, must provide a written statement to the contributor clearly stating the net amount of the contribution that is deductible. It must also contain an estimate of the value of the goods or services furnished by the charity to the person making the gift.

Deferred Giving

A person may commit today to make a gift of property to a charity in the future. The person making the gift does this by signing an agreement that declares the property will pass to the charity at a future date. Until that time, the person who made the future gift to the charity or some other person may receive the income from this property.

The person who makes a deferred gift will receive an income tax deduction in the year he or she makes the gift that equals the present value of the future interest given to charity.

Charitable Remainder Trust

One method of making a deferred gift to charity is through the charitable remainder trust. Such a trust is established in the same manner as any other trust. The terms of the trust define how much the beneficiary who is not the trustee will receive annually and for how long. The terms of the trust also provide that the charity is to become the beneficiary after a certain number of years. This designation of a charity as the ultimate beneficiary cannot be changed once the trust is signed. The charity must qualify as organizations described in Code Sections 170(c), 2055(a), and 2522(a) at the time of distribution in order for the income, estate, and gift tax charitable deductions to be available.

A charitable remainder trust is best used when a charitably inclined person owns appreciated property that he or she wishes to sell either to diversify or to produce a greater income stream. By contributing this property to a Charitable Remainder Trust, the person donating the property receives an immediate income tax deduction for the value of the charitable remainder. The trustee of the charitable remainder trust can sell this appreciated property and invest the entire net proceeds received from the sale. There will be no capital gains tax recognized by the charity since it is tax exempt.

There are two types of charitable remainder trusts. They are a charitable remainder annuity trust (CRAT) and a charitable remainder unitrust (CRUT). A significant difference between a charitable remainder annuity trust and a charitable remainder unitrust is the manner in which the income to the beneficiaries of these trusts is determined. A charitable remainder annuity trust provides for a fixed payout to be made no less often than annually to the income beneficiaries. The payout is a set-dollar amount, a fixed percentage or a fraction of the value of the initial contribution to the trust. The annual annuity payment must be at least five percent of the initial fair market value of the trust.

An example of a Charitable Remainder Annuity Trust is where a person contributes assets with a fair market value on the date of the gift equal to $1,000,000, to a Charitable Remainder Annuity Trust with an understanding that he or she or another specified person will receive a fifth of the amount contributed each year. The person donating the property or a specified person will receive $50,000 a year for his or her life.

This annual return is paid by the Trustee regardless of the investment performance of the trust assets. The return to the donor will not be affected by varying levels of income earned by the trust assets or by appreciation or depreciation in the market value of trust assets.

Similarly, a Charitable Remainder Unitrust (CRUT) distributes to a specified person at least once a year. However, the annual distribution is equal to a fixed percentage of the fair market value of the trust assets valued annually. While the percentage of the value of the trust assets to be received annually is fixed, the distribution will vary from year to year with the annual fair market value of the trust assets. Thus, the Charitable Remainder Unitrust protects the non-charitable lifetime beneficiary's cash flow from the effects of inflation. However, the Charitable Remainder Unitrust is more difficult to administer because the trust property must be revalued every year to calculate the unitrust payment amount.

An example of a Charitable Remainder Unitrust is where a person contributes assets with a fair market value on the date of gift equal to $1,000,000, to a Charitable Remainder Unitrust, and retains a right to receive five percent per year. The distribution in the first year will be $50,000. If the trust assets have increased to a market value of $1.5 million in 15 years, the distribution to the donor or the person designated by the donor will be $75,000 (5 percent x $1.5 million). If the trust assets have a market value of only $500,000 in year 15, the payout in that year will be $25,000 (5 percent of $500,000).

A Charitable Remainder Annuity Trust has only one method of payment. However, there are alternative methods for payment from a Charitable Remainder Unitrust.

In a Standard Charitable Remainder Unitrust (SCRUT), the income distributed to the donor or the designated beneficiary is determined by multiplying a fixed percentage times the value of the trust assets. The trust assets value is usually determined at the beginning of each year. This distribution to the income beneficiary is made regardless of the actual income earned by the trust assets. If the income is less than the amount necessary for distribution, the principal of the trust must be distributed to make up the shortfall.

In a Net Income Charitable Remainder Unitrust (NICRUT), the income beneficiary will receive the lesser of the standard unitrust distribution or the amount of the net income actually earned by the trust assets during the year. By example, the NICRUT may have been established with assets worth $1,000,000 and the trust may provide that the donor or the designated income beneficiary is to only receive 5 percent of asset value or trust net income for the year, whichever is less. If the income for the year is only $30,000, the income beneficiary will only receive $30,000, for that year.

By contrast, a Net Income With Make-up Charitable Remainder Unitrust (NIMCRUT) will permit the income beneficiary to establish a make-up account in an ensuing year when the trust net income is greater than the percentage amount. This means that in a subsequent year, a sufficient amount of income can be distributed from the trust to pay the entire year's income and to also pay the balance in the make-up account.

The present income tax deduction received by a donor contributing assets to a valid charitable remainder trust is determined by taking into consideration the fair market value of the property contributed to the trust, the term of the trust, the stated rate of the income, the frequency of payments, and the Internal Revenue Services discount rate in effect for the month of the gift. In the alternative, the discount rate in effect for either of the two months immediately preceding the gift established pursuant to Internal Revenue Code Section 7520 can be used. This is presently 120 percent of the federal mid-term rate, rounded to the nearest two-tenths of a percentage point. The federal mid-term rate is determined by computing the average market yield on obligations of the United States of America that have a maturity over three years and less than nine years.

Charitable Lead Trust

A Charitable Lead Trust provides that the charity is to receive an income stream for a fixed number of years or for the life or lives of an individual or individuals. At the end of this fixed term, the principal of the trust is returned to the donor or to an individual specified in the trust agreement. The donor may also be entitled to receive an income tax deduction for the value of the income stream that will be paid to the charity.

A Charitable Lead Trust must be irrevocable. However, the donor can retain the power to change the charity that is to receive the income interest.

The grantor of the Charitable Lead Trust is entitled to an income tax deduction only if the trust continues to be owned by the grantor. This means that the income earned on the trust will be taxed to the grantor. However, the grantor will receive a present income tax deduction in the year in which the trust is created. The income tax deduction is the present value of the expected income stream to charity. However, the trustee may invest in tax-exempt income producing assets. This means that the grantor will receive the immediate income tax deduction, but the annual income of the trust is tax-exempt.

Gift Annuities

A gift annuity is accomplished by gifting cash or other assets to a charity. In exchange, the charity agrees to pay an annuity payment to the donor. This agreement is not secured by any specific assets of the charity. It is important to remember that the person making the gift must report, as a capital gain, any appreciation on the property transferred in exchange for a gift annuity. However, this capital gain can be reported over the life expectancy of the person receiving the annuity.

The person contributing a gift annuity is entitled to an income tax deduction for a portion of the gift. The amount of this gift is determined by subtracting the present value of the stream of payments which will be received by the grantor from the present value of the property being contributed.

It is important to remember that the grantor's payments expire at his or her death. Accordingly, the amount contributed to the gift annuity will not be included in the grantor's estate for estate tax purposes.

Pooled Income Fund

Another form of creating a partial interest gift to charity is through the use of a pooled income fund. This is an arrangement created and managed by a charity. A person donates his or her assets to this trust, and these assets are pooled with other investors' assets. Each donor to this fund is entitled to receive a share of the annual net income earned on the trust assets. The income will vary each year on the basis of the investment performance of the pooled fund. The investor's share in the trust assets is paid to the charity when the investor dies. The person contributing to the pooled income fund receives a charitable deduction for the present value of the interest that is expected to be received by the charity on the death of the contributor. The amount of this charitable deduction depends, in part, on how much income the donor expects to receive annually.

CHAPTER 31

PROBATE

- Personal Representative's Compensation
- Attorney Fees
- Alternatives to Formal Probate
- Summary Administration
- Disposition Without Need of Administration
- Automobile
- Homestead

The purpose of probate is to collect a deceased person's assets; pay his or her claims, taxes, and administrative expenses from these assets; and distribute the remainder of the assets after administrative expenses to the beneficiaries entitled to receive them. A personal representative (known as an executor) is appointed by the court to pay the deceased's claims and taxes and to distribute the remainder of the estate assets according to the terms of the deceased person's will. If a person dies without a valid will, the personal representative then distributes the remainder of the estate assets in fixed percentages to the heirs named in the Florida statute.

A personal representative appointed by a Florida court must take possession of all the deceased's personal property no matter where it is located. The Florida personal representative also assumes the responsibility for administering the deceased's real property in this state with the exception of the homestead. Since the Florida courts have no jurisdiction over real property outside the boundaries of the state, the Florida personal representative does not have the authority to control the administration or management of real property in another state. Instead, the beneficiaries of that real property in another state must request that the court where the real property is located appoint a personal representative. This is called an ancillary administration.

A claim must be filed against the estate of the deceased person in the probate proceeding within the latter of three months after notice to creditors was first published or 30 days after the personal representative notifies a known creditor.

A personal representative has the authority to represent the interests of all persons affected by the estate proceeding. Since a creditor of a deceased person cannot make a claim against a person who owes the deceased money, it is the responsibility of the personal representative to take steps to collect the deceased's assets, not just for the beneficiaries but also for the deceased's creditors.

Personal Representative's Compensation

The personal representative is entitled to receive compensation from the estate assets for his or her services. The Florida statutes provide that a certain commission will be assumed reasonable for ordinary services rendered to an estate by the personal representative. This commission is based on the value of the probate assets and any income those assets earn. The commission is calculated as follows:

1. at the rate of 3 percent for the first $1 million
2. at the rate of 2.5 percent for all above $1 million and not exceeding $5 million
3. at the rate of 2 percent for all above $5 million and not exceeding $10 million
4. at the rate of 1.5 percent for all above $10 million.

In addition to this commission, a personal representative may be allowed additional compensation for extraordinary services, including:

1. the sale of real or personal property
2. bringing suit for the estate
3. adjusting or paying taxes
4. carrying on the deceased's business

The compensation for ordinary services (or for extraordinary services) may be increased or decreased by the court. To determine whether to do this for such services, the court must consider these factors:

1. the promptness, efficiency and skill with which the administration was handled by the personal representative
2. the responsibilities assumed and the potential liabilities of the personal representative
3. whether the estate benefited or suffered from the personal representatives services
4. whether the administration of this service was complex or simple

Attorney Fees

The attorney for the personal representative is also compensated from the estate assets for his or her services. Florida has a statute that allows for reasonable compensation for services provided to an estate by the personal representative's attorney. This compensation for the attorney in a formal estate administration that is presumed to be reasonable is based upon the value of the assets and all income earned. The compensation that is presumed to be reasonable is computed as follows:

1. $1,500 for estates having a value of $40,000 or less
2. an additional $750 for estates having a value of more than $40,000 and not exceeding $70,000
3. an additional $750 for estates having a value of more than $70,000 and not exceeding $100,000
4. for estates having a value in excess of $100,000, at the rate of 3 percent on any amount above this up to $1,000,000
5. at the rate of 2.5 percent for all above $1 million and not exceeding $3 million
6. at the rate of 2 percent for all above $3 million and not exceeding $5 million
7. at the rate of 1.5 percent for all above $5 million and not exceeding $10 million
8. at the rate of 1 percent for all above $10 million

This "presumed reasonable" statute does not prohibit the attorney and the personal representative from entering into another method for compensation for the attorney. In addition to reasonable compensation for ordinary services, the attorney for the personal representative is allowed reasonable compensation for an extraordinary service, including the purchase or sale of real property by the personal representative, involvement in a will contest or a will interpretation, a proceeding for determination of beneficiaries, a contested claim, a petition for apportionment of estate taxes or any litigation by or against the estate.

The attorney is also entitled to compensation for preparation of the estate's federal estate tax return. Once the gross estate is determined and the return is prepared by the attorney, a fee of one-half of 1 percent of the value up to $10 million and one-fourth of 1 percent of the value in excess of $10 million of the gross estate is considered reasonable compensation for attorney's services.

The compensation for ordinary services or for extraordinary services may be increased or decreased by the court, in which case the court considers the same factors it does in deciding whether to adjust the amount of compensation for a personal representative.

Alternatives to Formal Probate

There are times when the value of a deceased person's estate does not warrant a formal probate administration. These instances are as follows:

Summary Administration

The circuit judge is authorized to grant a summary administration when the fair market value of property subject to probate administration does not exceed $75,000. An order of summary administration may also be obtained to confirm the title for a protected homestead passing to a surviving spouse or to an heir-at-law, regardless of its value. A protected homestead is the decedent's residence where he or she intended to permanently reside at the time of his or her death. A summary administration is also allowed for a protected homestead because the deceased's creditor claims cannot attach to this real property.

If a petition for summary administration for assets presently having a value of less than $75,000, or for assets exempt from creditor claims, is filed with the clerk of the court by all the beneficiaries and the surviving spouse, the circuit judge may order immediate distribution of this property to the beneficiaries named in the will. An order of summary administration will not be granted by the circuit judge if the decedent has known creditors which the beneficiaries have not agreed to pay. An exception is when no creditor timely files a claim after receiving notice of the opportunity to file a claim and the three-month period has passed since a notice to creditors was published. Another exception would be if the two-year statute of limitations for creditors to file claims has expired.

Disposition without Need of Administration

The Florida statutes allow for the distribution of a deceased's assets without probate when the value of the deceased's nonexempt assets does not exceed the preferred funeral expense of $6,000 and the reasonable and necessary medical and hospital expenses of the last 60 days of the deceased's last illness. If the circuit judge is satisfied after reviewing the petition and the copies of the attached receipts for the paid funeral and medical expenses, the judge may authorize the payment of the proceeds of the bank accounts to the person who paid those expenses.

Automobile

If there is no need for probate except for the disposition of an automobile, the beneficiary named in the deceased's last will and testament can apply at the county tax collector's office for the Florida Department of Motor Vehicles to issue a new motor vehicle certificate of title in the name of the beneficiary.

If a person died without a last will and testament, an heir of the deceased owner can apply to the Department of Motor Vehicles for a new certificate of title with an affidavit that the estate of the deceased is not indebted and the surviving spouse and the heirs have amicably agreed to this title transfer.

Homestead

The Florida Constitution prohibits the devise of a deceased's homestead if he or she is survived by a spouse or minor child. The Florida statutes then state that the surviving spouse is to receive a life estate and the deceased's descendants who are alive at the time of the deceased's death receive a vested remainder interest in the homestead. If there are no surviving lineal descendents, the surviving spouse receives the entire interest in the homestead. This statute has created a hardship for the surviving spouse who must pay the taxes and the homeowner's insurance and the lineal descendents are required to pay the principal payments on the mortgage installments. Further, there was no provision in the statute permitting the surviving spouse to sell her life estate without the joinder of the lineal descendents. In addition, a child who was known as a remainderman could not force a sale of the homestead. Fortunately, there is new legislation that became effective October 1, 2010, that permits a spouse to elect to receive an undivided one-half interest in the homestead as a tenant in common with the lineal descendents. However, it is important to remember that this election must be made by the surviving spouse within six months after the death of the spouse. The statute requires the election to be timely filed in the official records of the Clerk of the Court where the property is situate. If the election is timely filed, then the surviving spouse will be able to ask the lineal descendents to pay one-half of the insurance and taxes. If they refuse, the surviving spouse can ask the court to order the property to be sold if it is not capable of partition.

An exception to the Florida homestead act relates to a homestead that is owned with a spouse as tenants by the entirety. In that event, the homestead automatically survives solely by operation of law to the surviving spouse without probate. Likewise, it is important to remember that a spouse may sign a valid prenuptial or post nuptial agreement waiving any survivorship interest in the homestead. This is further explained in chapter 27.

The constitutional prohibition on a parent devising a homestead if he or she was survived by a minor child also brought about an unwanted result where the homestead received by a minor child had to be managed by a guardian of the property. The homestead could not be devised to a trustee. This often resulted in the unnecessary expense related to the annual cost of a guardian of the property, his or her attorney fees and a guardianship accounting. In recognition of this problem, the legislature passed a new statute that became effective

October 1, 2010. This new statute permits the owner to convey his or her homestead during lifetime to an irrevocable homestead trust. The provisions of the homestead trust permit the trustee to manage the homestead after the owner's death for the minor child until he or she attains at least age 18. The owner of the homestead can still retain a life estate use of the real property. Thus, there is no loss of the save-our-homes homestead tax exclusion of the homestead exemption against creditors. The owner can still retain in the trust provision the power to alter the beneficiaries of the trust during the owner's lifetime, so long as he does not direct the ownership to the owner or his creditors or his estate. Thus, the owner can still exclude a child from inheriting the property even after the property is conveyed to the revocable trust. Retention of the power to alter the beneficial use of the property will cause the property to not be immediately taxed as a gift.

CHAPTER 32

ARRANGING THE FUNERAL

- Pre-Need Arrangements
- Cremation
- The Need for Written Funeral Instructions
- Organ Donation

Pre-Need Arrangements

Coming to terms with a loved one's death is difficult enough without also having to make the funeral arrangements. That is why it is important for a person to express in advance his or her desire concerning the type of funeral and the method for disposing of the remains.

Most funeral homes now offer assistance with prearranging a funeral. Counselors will discuss all aspects of the goods and services to be provided. A person can select in advance exactly what type of service he or she prefers, whether he or she desires to be buried or cremated, and where he or she will be interred. Advance planning will also avoid emotional overspending by your family.

A prepaid burial and funeral agreement is a hedge against rising costs. The Florida legislature has recognized that the cost of funerals has risen by increasing the preferred claim for a burial in a probate proceeding to $6,000.

A pre-need funeral provider must be licensed through the Florida Department of Banking and Finance. The state of Florida will require financial statements demonstrating solvency of the licensed funeral director and licensed funeral home. The funeral director must establish a trust account with a bank in Florida where the purchaser's funds are deposited, and the account will be subject to audit every three years or less.

Any money paid in advance of a pre-need funeral arrangement is trusted - that is, placed on deposit in a reputable bank. There is a 30 day right-to-rescind any preneed contract, and the purchaser has the right to receive most of his or her purchase price back if the contract is canceled. Since there are different statutes governing funeral home and cemetery trusting, the refund will differ between funeral homes and cemeteries.

A funeral director offering merchandise for sale to a prospective purchaser must comply with the following requirements:

1. The least expensive casket offered for sale must be displayed in the same general manner that the other caskets are displayed.

2. The funeral director must not discourage a customer's purchase of any funeral merchandise or service that was advertised for sale with the purpose of encouraging additional purchases of more expensive merchandise or services.

3. The sale price of all caskets displayed for sale must be clearly marked, whether displayed on location or in books, brochures, and catalogs.

If information about the merchandise and services offered by a funeral home is requested by telephone, the response regarding the retail prices of funeral merchandise and services must be accurate. A funeral director must make a full disclosure of all services and merchandise available to the customer prior to selection.

A funeral director must also fully explain to the customer the legal requirements concerning the handling of the body, especially concerning the type of casket or container required. The customer should be given a complete explanation of the pricing alternatives, such as those for graveside services, direct disposition, and the donation of the body without any rites or ceremonies, prior to the delivery of the body.

A funeral director must have available for the customer a complete, updated list of all retail prices for any number of items or services that the director regularly offers for sale. Such items include the cost for the transfer of the body to the funeral home; embalming (along with the statement that embalming is not required by state law); the cost for the use of facilities for viewing and for the funeral service; the use of hearse, limousine, or other transportation; and the alternative-container price ranges. The statement presented to the customer must include the name, address, and phone number of the funeral home and a statement that the customer may limit his or her choice to particular items. The customer must be advised that he or she will be charged for only those items selected. It should also be noted that there may be an extra charge for other items such as a cemetery fee and flowers.

The funeral director must furnish to the customer a written agreement listing the prices and items discussed while making funeral arrangements. This will include specifically itemized cash advances. Once completed to the satisfaction of the customers and according to Florida state statute, the document must be signed by each party and dated.

Cremation

Should a family wish to cremate the remains of a loved one, the following is required:

1. a written authorization from the next of kin.

2. a signed death certificate
3. the medical examiner's authorization (which may require a $25 fee)
4. a permit from the county health department
5. a waiting period of 48 hours after death

The Need for Written Funeral Instructions

In a recent Florida case, the mother of a deceased daughter appealed the trial judge's decision to award the right to dispose of her daughter's remains to the guardian for the granddaughter's only living minor child. The trial judge based his decision on the statute governing state medical examiners. This statute states that in the event more than one legally authorized person claims a body in the custody of the medical examiner for interment, the request of the surviving spouse makes the decision. If there is no surviving spouse, this statute states the lineal descendents of the deceased make the decision. A parent only has the right to make this decision if there is no spouse or lineal descendent. The trial court noted that the mother would have the preference if the body had been at a funeral home. This is because the statute governing funeral homes states if there is no written instruction to the contrary and there is no spouse or child over 18 years, the parent makes the decision.

The Appeals court ruled that neither the medical examiner statute or the funeral home statute applied to the outcome of this case because the suit involved private parties engaged in a pre-burial dispute over the remains. Otherwise stated, the trial court was not being asked to consider whether a funeral home or medical examiner was liable for its decision regarding the disposition of the remains.

The court instead stated that the common law applied. The court held that in absence of a testamentary disposition, the spouse of the decedent or the next of kin has the right to the possession of the body for burial or other lawful disposition. However, the court of appeals also recognized that a written testamentary disposition is not conclusive of the decedent's intent if it can be shown by clear and convincing evidence that he intended another disposition for his body. Thus, a person has a right to subsequently change his or her mind regarding the disposition of his or her body despite having previously stated a contrary preference in a will.

The court of appeals did not overrule the trial judge's decision despite his having applied the wrong law because the deceased's last wish with respect to the disposition of her remains was to be buried in the Bahamas next to her deceased son and the Guardian of her minor child stated an intention to honor that wish.

This case brings to forefront that a good estate plan should specify in the last will and testament or in the funeral director's prearrangement forms how a person's body should be disposed. Any subsequent contrary decision should be clarified in a codicil to the will or an amendment to the prearrangement forms. Without such preplanning, this case demonstrates the potential for unnecessary expense and delays attributed to litigation over the disposition of a person's remains.

Organ Donation

The Florida statutes state that a person may make a gift of his or her body or body parts which will be effective after death. The donation of all or part of his or her body must be for the purpose of tissue and organ preservation or transplanting or for medical research. The Florida statutes permit a donation of a gift of a body or parts of a body for only these purposes to:

1. any hospital, surgeon, or physician for medical or dental education or research, advancement of medical or dental science, therapy, or transplantation, any accredited medical or dental school, college, or university for education research, advancement of medical or dental science, or therapy
2. any bank or storage facility for medical or dental education, research advancement of medical or dental science, therapy, or transplantation
3. any individual specified by name for therapy or transplantation needed by him or her

There can be no restriction on the possible recipient of such an anatomical gift on the basis of race, color, religion, sex, national origin, age, physical handicap, health status, marital status, or economic status. Any such restriction is unenforceable.

Florida's Agency for Health Care Administration and the Department of Highway Safety and Motor Vehicles have implemented a registry which records organ and tissue donations submitted through the driver license identification program and by other sources. There are 6,926,821 Florida residents who are registered organ or tissue donors as of December 31, 2012. This registry permits access to this information only by accredited hospitals, organ and tissue procurement agencies, and other parties identified by the agency as having a need for this information.

A person may make an anatomical gift as part of the process of obtaining or renewing a driver's license or through programs established by the Florida Agency for Health Care Administration. The Florida Department of Highway Safety and Motor Vehicles will then indicate the individual's intent to donate organs or tissues on the front of his or her driver license. Further information regarding this program and the organ donor form can be found on the Internet at www.hsmv.state.fl.us. Additional information may also be obtained by contacting the Agency for Health Care Administration on the Internet at otdonors@fdhc. state.fl.us.

Another way a gift of all or part of the body for the purpose of tissue and organ preservation or transplanting or for medical research may be made is through a will. The gift becomes effective upon the death of the person who made the will without waiting for probate. If the will is not probated or if it is declared invalid, the gift of the body is nevertheless valid to the extent that it was relied upon in good faith.

An anatomical gift may also be made by a document other than a will. The document must be signed in the presence of two witnesses who must also sign the document in the donor's presence. If the donor cannot sign, the document may be signed at the donor's direction and in his or her presence and the presence of two witnesses who must sign the document in the donor's presence.

If an anatomical gift is not made through a program established by the Department of Highway Safety and Motor Vehicles or the Agency for Health Care Administration and is made by a person to a specific donee such as a medical college, the document, other than a will, may be delivered to the donee to expedite the appropriate procedures immediately after death. However, delivery of the document before death is not necessary for the gift to be valid.

A donor may amend or revoke an anatomical gift at any time before death by signing and delivering a statement to the proposed donee of the anatomical gift. The Florida statutes also permit a person to notify the Department of Highway Safety and Motor Vehicles that he or she has withdrawn his or her gift of organs or tissues. In such event, the Department is required to update its registry noting the withdrawal.

An amendment or revocation of an anatomical gift may also be made by an oral statement that is made to a spouse. Such an amendment or revocation of an anatomical gift may also be made by an oral statement that is made in the presence of two persons and communicated to the family or attorney of the person intending to make the anatomical gift or to the donee of the anatomical gift. An anatomical gift may also be amended or revoked by a statement during a terminal illness addressed to an attending physician or a signed document found on the donor's person or in the donor's effects. An anatomical gift made by will may also be amended or revoked in the manner provided by law for the amendment or revocation of a will.

The Florida statutes state that if a decedent signed an agreement concerning an anatomical gift, his or her health care surrogate may carry out the instructions. The Florida statutes also state that if a decedent has not executed an agreement concerning an anatomical gift or designated a surrogate to make anatomical gifts, a member of one of the classes of persons listed below, in order of priority stated and in absence of actual notice of contrary indications by the decedent or actual notice of opposition by a member of the same or prior class, may give all or any part of the decedent's body as an anatomical gift:

1. the spouse of the decedent;
2. an adult son or daughter of the decedent;
3. either parent of the decedent;
4. an adult brother or sister of the decedent;
5. a grandparent of the decedent;
6. a guardian of the person of the decedent at the time of his or her death.

In addition, a court of competent jurisdiction may appoint a representative ad litem for the purpose of making an anatomical gift if the representative ad litem ascertains that no person of higher priority exists who objects to the gift of all or any part of the decedent's body and that no evidence exists of the decedent having made a communication expressing a desire that his or her body or body parts not be donated upon death.

The Florida statutes also state that no anatomical gift may be made by a spouse if any adult son or daughter objects. The statutes also require that those of higher priority, if they are reasonably available, must be contacted and made aware of the proposed gift.

The Florida statutes provide that after removal of the donated organs or tissues, the remainder of the body vests in the surviving spouse, next of kin or other person under obligation to dispose of the body.

CHAPTER 33

VETERANS' BENEFITS

- Overview of Veterans' Benefits
- Compensation
- Non-Service Connected Pension
- Medical Care
- Geriatric Services
- Prescription Benefits

Overview of Veterans' Benefits

A person who has served in the United States Armed Forces may be entitled to receive compensation from the Veterans' Administration for service-connected disabilities that occurred or were aggravated during a period of military service. A veteran may also be entitled to receive a non-service connected pension. In addition, a veteran may be entitled to receive health care services from the Veterans Health Administration that is a branch of the Veterans' Administration. This department is separate from the Veterans' Benefits Administration. It is important to remember that a person is not automatically entitled to medical care because he or she is a veteran. The Veterans' Health Administration's medical care is primarily related to medical care for health problems that occurred as a result of military service. Also, a veteran must not have been dishonorably discharged in order to receive benefits.

Compensation

Veterans' compensation is based on an impairment of earning capability that is related to a service-connected disability. It is important to remember that the disability does not have to be related to combat. VA compensation and pension benefits cost of living allowance (COLA) is paid based on the Social Security Administration (SSA) COLA. This year (2015) SSA did increase the COLA. The 2015 Veterans' Administration compensation rate for a veteran who is not married with a 10 percent disability rating is $133.17 per month. The Veterans Administration compensation rate for a veteran who is not married with a 100 percent disability rating is $2,906.83 per month. A veteran may be eligible for an increased or a special monthly compensation that may be greater than these amounts if the veteran is in need of aid and attendance of another to care for him or her. The Veterans Administration may re-evaluate a service-connected condition. If the extent of the disability has increased or decreased, the percentage of disability may be changed.

Non-Service Connected Pension

A non-service connected pension is available each month to a permanent and totally disabled veteran and his or her spouse or dependent when the veteran is 65 years or older, honorably discharged after at least 90 days of active duty with one day being during a wartime, and experiencing financial need. This benefit is also available to the surviving spouse of a deceased wartime veteran. There is no requirement that the veteran over age 65 prove that his or his spouse is actually disabled. It is presumed that because the age of the veteran is over 65 that the veteran is disabled. A veteran who is younger than age 65 must demonstrate that he or she is permanently and totally disabled in order to receive this financial assistance. This disability for a person under age 65 must be an impairment that renders it impossible for the average person to follow a substantially gainful occupation. This impairment must be one that is reasonably certain to continue throughout life.

There are three types of monthly non-service connected pensions that are paid by the Veterans Administration to offset the cost of necessary health care. They are called Low Income Pension, Housebound Benefits and Aid and Attendance benefits. An extra benefit amount is if the claimant is "permanently housebound." This is demonstrated by the person being substantially confined to his or her dwelling and that this condition will continue throughout his or her lifetime. More income is available to a person who is confined to assisted living due to medical reasons giving rise to an inability to perform at least two activities of daily living.

It is not necessary that the veteran have been in combat or even in the country where the war was fought to receive these benefits. In general, wartime is considered the period of World War I, World War II (December 7, 1941 - December 31, 1946), the Korean War (June 27, 1950 - January 1, 1955), Vietnam War (August 5, 1964 - May 7, 1975), and the Gulf War (August 2, 1990 through a date to be set by law by Presidential Proclamation). However, anyone who enlists after September 7, 1980 generally has to have served at least 24 months or the full period for which a person was called or ordered to active duty in order to receive any benefits based on that period of service.

Once the disability and wartime service test is met, the veteran or his or her spouse must meet a three part means test qualification before receiving a VA pension. Two components of the means test are the veteran and his or her spouse's gross income and net worth.

The third aspect is determining the allowable deductions from gross income in order to compute income for VA purposes.

First, the payments to the potential claimant, his or her spouse, and dependent children from all sources are considered. This includes recurring income such as social security and pensions, as well as irregular income for the next twelve months. The unreimbursed medical expenses are then excluded from income. Unreimbursed medical expenses include but are not limited to Medicare Part B, Medigap premiums and Medicare Part D premiums and prescription drug payments as well as caregiver expenses or recurring assisted living expenses. The gross income less the unreimbursed medical expenses will determine the claimant's Income for VA Purposes (IVAP). The goal is for the IVAP to be $0. This is because there is a reduction against the Monthly Maximum Pension Rate (the income limit) for every dollar of IVAP.

The Projected Maximum Monthly Annual Pension Rate (the Income Limit) for 2015

Wartime Veteran

Type of Benefit	Monthly Maximum Annual Pension Rate
Service Pension	$1,072
Housebound	$1,310
Aid and Attendance	$1,788

Surviving Spouse

Type of Benefit	Monthly Maximum Annual Pension Rate
Death Pension	$ 719
Housebound	$ 879
Aid and Attendance	$1,149

The veteran's net worth is also a factor in determining eligibility for improved pension. The term net worth for VA purposes includes all property owned by the claimant and his or her spouse, except for a personal residence, personal effects and an automobile for personal use. Assets exceeding $80,000 will normally be found to be sufficient for a person to be able to support himself or herself and the spouse. However, net worth below $80,000 could still be a bar. Countable assets for a couple of $40,000 and $20,000 for an individual are normally found to be reasonable. This test is subjective depending on the age of the applicant. Presently, assets may be gifted by the applicant before applying for assistance. However, legislation is being considered to penalize applicants who make gifts to become qualified for assistance. It is important to remember that gifted assets will disqualify an applicant and his or her spouse for Medicaid purposes for a period of ineligibility if gifted within five years of applying for Medicaid assistance. Also, the pension benefit is reduced to $90 a month if the veteran is in a nursing home and being provided Medicaid services.

Medical Care

The Veterans Administration does provide health care services to veterans. These include hospital care at a Veterans Administration medical center and nursing home care at a Veterans Administration nursing center. However, a veteran is required to make a co-payment that is based on the inpatient Medicare deductible rate, which is adjusted annually. These co-payment rates are explained in Chapter 2 of this book. In order to receive these health care benefits, the veteran must be enrolled in the Veterans Administrations health care system. Nursing home care is not provided to all enrolled veterans. Nursing home care is only provided to veterans needing nursing home care for a service-related condition to veterans with a service-connected disability rating of 70 percent or more and veterans who have a service-connected disability of 60 percent and are unemployable. There are also state-run veteran nursing homes. The VA provides funds to states to help them build the homes and pays a portion of the costs for veterans eligible for VA health care. The states, however, set eligibility criteria for admission. A service-connected disability is a disability that the Veterans Administration has officially ruled was incurred or aggravated while on active duty in the military and in the line of duty. When the Veterans Administration rules that the illness or condition is directly related to active military service, a disability rating is assigned.

Geriatric Services

An enrolled veteran may also be entitled to receive certain geriatric services. He or she may receive either an inpatient or outpatient evaluation of a veteran's ability to care for his or her therapeutic day care programs that provide medical and rehabilitation services; respite care; nursing, physical therapy, and other services provided in the veteran's home and hospice and palliative care.

Prescription Benefits

Prescription co-payments are charged only for outpatient treatment. There is no difference in cost between generic and name brand medication. The co-pay is $8 for Priority Groups 2 through 6 for each formulary 30-day or less supply of medication and a co-pay of $9 for Priority Groups 7-8 for each formulary 30-day or less supply of medication. However, there is no co-pay charged for a veteran who is 50 percent disabled or more with a service-connected disability; a veteran who has been determined unemployable due to his service-connected conditions; a veteran who needs medication to treat a specific service-connected disability; a former Prisoner of War and a veteran whose income is below the maximum annual rate for a Veterans Administration pension. If a veteran decides to participate in the Medicare plan, his or her Veteran Administration prescription drug coverage will not be affected by the Medicare Prescription Drug Act. This is because the Veteran Administrations prescription drug coverage is considered creditable coverage. If a veteran disenrolls or loses his or her Veterans Administration Drug coverage, the veteran will generally have 62 days to sign up for a Medicare plan without being subject to a penalty.

Chapter 34

Veterans' Cemeteries

• Veterans' Cemeteries

In 1862, President Lincoln signed legislation authorizing the establishment of national cemeteries for the soldiers who die in the service of the country. Fourteen cemeteries were established in that year. These national cemeteries were the beginning of what has become the National Cemetery System.

Burial in a national cemetery is based on military service. There is no charge for burial in a national cemetery. Today, there are 144 national veterans' cemeteries in the United States. Three active veterans' cemeteries are located in Florida at Pensacola and Bushnell for casketed or cremated remains and at Bay Pines for cremation burials only.

A veteran may choose to be buried in any active cemetery along with his or her spouse and dependent child. There is a cost savings in choosing a veterans' cemetery. The veteran is entitled to a gravesite, the opening and closing of the grave, a headstone and the perpetual care of the gravesite. The U.S. Department of Veterans Affairs also furnishes at no expense to the next of kin the grave liners for a new grave in national cemeteries that have space available.

Some of these veterans' cemeteries have a special area for cremated remains. Such remains are interred in an in-ground gravesite or placed in a garden niche or in a columbarium, where available. Many national cemeteries have also set aside suitable areas to commemorate veterans whose remains were not recovered or identified, were buried at sea, or are otherwise unavailable for internment.

Surviving spouses are also entitled to a burial site until remarriage. If the remarriage ends through the death of or divorce from the new spouse, though, the veteran's spouse may still choose a burial in the national cemetery where the veteran is buried. There are no reserved gravesites. They are available on a first-come, first-served basis.

Headstones and markers are inscribed with the name of the deceased veteran's year of birth and death and the deceased's branch of service. The headstone may also include the deceased's rank, war service, preferred religious emblem, and a list of valor and purple heart awards received. If the remains are not available for burial, a headstone or marker can be placed in memory of the deceased. Flat bronze, granite or marble grave markers and upright marble or granite headstones are available to mark graves in the style consistent with existing monuments at the national cemetery. A United States flag is usually provided by a funeral director to drape the casket or accompany the urn of a veteran.

If the veteran's death is service-connected, the spouse is entitled to reimbursement of the cost of transportation of the body to the national cemetery nearest the veteran's last place of residence, provided burial space is available. The spouse of a veteran whose death is service-connected is also reimbursed for the funeral and burial expenses in connection with the death up to $2,000.

If the death was not service-connected but the veteran was receiving a monthly veteran disability benefit at the time of death, the spouse is entitled to be reimbursed up to $300 for burial and funeral expenses at a national cemetery. This burial benefit is also available if a veteran dies in a VA facility or a nursing home under a VA contract. Should the veteran be buried elsewhere, only a $300 plot allowance is allowed.

CHAPTER 35

THE PATIENT PROTECTION AND AFFORDABLE CARE ACT

- Overview of the Patient and Affordable Care Act
- Young Adult Coverage
- Unlimited Coverage
- Pre-Existing Condition
- Non-Rescission
- Non-Discrimination
- Required Coverage
- Penalty
- The Health Insurance Exchange
- Premium Tax Credit
- Legal Challenges to the Affordable Care Act

Overview of the Patient and Affordable Care Act

There were 51.5 million uninsured nonelderly United States citizens in 2010. The Patient Protection and Affordable Care Act was enacted to ensure that all Americans have access to quality, affordable health care. The Congressional Budget Office has determined that this law could provide health insurance coverage to as many as 94% of the presently uninsured Americans. The Patient Protection and Affordable Care Act became effective when it was signed into law by President Barack Obama on March 30, 2010. Group health insurance plans in existence as of March 30, 2010, may remain as they are written. A few of the important provisions of this new law that became effective in 2010 are set forth in the following paragraphs.

Young Adult Coverage

Group health plans and health insurers offering group or individual health insurance with dependent child coverage must make available optional coverage for the enrollee's dependent adult children who are younger than age 26. The coverage must be provided even if the child is married or disabled. The child does not have to be a student.

Unlimited Coverage

Group health plans and health insurers offering group or individual health insurance may not impose limits on benefits or caps. The new rules are not construed in preventing the coverage from imposing an annual or lifetime per beneficiary cap on specific covered benefits that are not considered "essential health benefits."

Pre-Existing Condition

Beginning in 2014, this Act ended the medical underwriting and pre-existing condition exclusions. Insurers are prohibited from denying coverage or setting rates based on health status, medical condition, claims experience, genetic information, evidence of domestic violence, or other health-related factors. Deductibles in the small group market will not be allowed to exceed $2,000 for an individual and $4,000 for a family.

Non-Rescission

Group health plans and health insurers offering group or individual health insurance may not rescind an insured's coverage once it is issued, except for fraud or intentional misrepresentation of material facts. Such coverage may not be cancelled without prior notice to the enrollee. However, mandatory renewal or continued coverage is not required if premiums are not paid or are paid untimely or that type of coverage is no longer provided in the market.

Non-Discrimination

The health insurance benefits provided to highly compensated employees must be provided to all other employees. However, the group insurance plan can exclude employees who have not completed three years of service or who are part-time or who are under 25 years of age.

Required Coverage

The Affordable Care Act initially required nearly every resident of the United States to obtain minimum health insurance coverage by January 1, 2014 or to be exempt. The deadline was extended to March 31, 2014. Minimum essential coverage is not required the individual and his or her dependent(s) covered under either Medicare Part A, Medicaid, the Child Health Insurance Program, Tricare, Veteran's heath care, an employer sponsored plan, an individual plan or the Health and Human Services' plan or a state risk pool.

The Penalty

Taxpayers who earn more than the amount required to file a federal income tax return are subject to a shared responsibility payment if they do not have the minimum essential health insurance coverage. Under these provisions, a taxpayer is potentially liable for not having required health insurance coverage for him or herself, and for any individual the taxpayer could claim as a dependent for federal income tax purposes. Thus, all children generally must have minimum essential coverage or qualify for a coverage exemption for each month in the year. Otherwise, the primary taxpayer or taxpayers who can claim the child as a dependent for federal income tax purposes will also owe an individual shared responsibility payment for the child if the child is not covered by health insurance.

People who do not comply with the individual coverage requirement will be charged a penalty, assessed through the Internal Revenue Code. Exemptions from that requirement or its associated penalties are provided for several categories of people including those with taxable income below the 2014 threshold for mandatory tax filing of a federal income tax which is $10,150 for a single filer under age 65 or $11,700 for a single filer age 65 or older and $20,300 for a married couple both under age 65 and $21,500 for a married couple if either is over age 65 in 2014, unauthorized immigrants, members of certain religious groups, people who would have to pay more than 8 percent of their income for health insurance, prisoners, and those who obtain a hardship waiver.

The penalty for 2014 is equal to the greater of 1 percent of the household income that is above the tax return filing threshold for the taxpayer's filing status, or the family's flat dollar amount, which is $95 per adult and $47.50 per child (under age 18), limited to a family maximum of $285. The shared responsibility payment is capped at the national average premium for a bronze level qualified health plan available through the Marketplace in 2014 that would cover everyone in the taxpayer's household who does not have coverage and does not qualify for a coverage exemption. The penalty increases in 2015 to 2 percent of household income that is above the tax return filing threshold and the flat dollar amount increases to $325 per adult and $162.50 per child. The penalty increases in 2016 to 2.5 percent of household income of the household income that is above the tax return filing threshold and the flat dollar amount increases to $695 per adult and $347.50 per child. After 2016, the flat dollar amounts may increase with inflation.

The Health Insurance Exchange

The Affordable Care Act also creates the Health Insurance Marketplace, also known as the Marketplace or the Exchange. The Marketplace is where taxpayers find information about health insurance options, purchase qualified health plans and, if eligible, obtain help paying premiums and out-of-pocket costs. A new tax credit, the premium tax credit, is available only if the taxpayer purchased a qualified health plan through the Marketplace. This credit helps eligible taxpayers pay for coverage.

Premium Tax Credit

Taxpayers who purchase a qualified health plan from a health Insurance Marketplace may be eligible for the premium tax credit. This federal tax credit helps eligible taxpayers pay for health insurance premiums. When enrolling in a qualified health plan through the Marketplace, eligible taxpayers may choose to have some or all of the benefit of the credit paid in advance to their insurance company as advance credit payments or wait to claim all of the benefit of the premium tax credit on their tax return. Taxpayers must file a tax return to claim the premium tax credit. In general, taxpayers are allowed a premium tax credit if the taxpayer's income is at least 100 percent but not more than 400 percent of the federal poverty level for the taxpayer's family size.

Legal Challenges to Affordable Care Act

First Challenge

The Affordable Care Act was the subject of a Constitutional challenge that was decided by the United States Supreme Court in 2012. The government contended that this individual mandate (to buy health insurance) was within Congress' power because the failure to purchase insurance has a substantial and deleterious effect on interstate commerce. The majority of the members of the U.S. Supreme Court held that the Congress does not have the authority to order people to buy health insurance. This is because the commerce clause of our U.S. Constitution presupposes the existence of commercial activity. The court found that individuals were not engaging in commerce by declining to buy an unwanted insurance product. Instead, the act would compel individuals to become active in commerce by purchasing the insurance product.

While the court ruled that a person cannot be compelled to buy health insurance, the U.S. Supreme Court did hold that beginning in 2014, those who did not comply with the mandate to buy health insurance will have to pay the "shared responsibility payment" tax explained above. It is estimated that some four million citizens each year will choose to pay the IRS rather than buy insurance.

The second provision of the Affordable Care Act directly challenged in this case was Medicaid expansion. The original Medicaid program was designed to cover medical services for four particular categories of the needy: the disabled, the blind, the elderly and needy families with dependent children. The Affordable Care Act would expand the scope of the Medicaid program and increase the number of individuals a state must cover. For example, the Act required state programs to provide Medicaid coverage in 2015 to the entire nonelderly population with incomes below 133% of the poverty level. The poverty limit for an individual in 2015 is $11,670.

It is projected that Medicaid will be expanded to include about 17 million additional people in the United States. The Act provided additional federal funding to cover the States' costs in expanding this Medicaid coverage. For instance, the Act stated that the Federal Government will pay 100 percent of the cost of covering these newly eligible individuals though 2016. In the following years, the federal payment level will gradually decrease to a minimum of 90 percent of the cost of the expanded coverage.

The new law provided that if a state did not expand its Medicaid coverage, Congress could deprive a state of its existing Medicaid funding for the needy. However, the U.S. Supreme Court ruled that the federal government cannot effectively coerce states into accepting the Medicaid expansion by withdrawing all of a state's present Medicaid funding if it refuses to expand its Medicaid coverage. Accordingly, the U.S. Supreme Court held that a state can decide to opt out of the expansion of Medicaid services without losing its current Medicaid funding for the needy presently being served. The U.S. Supreme Court also ruled that since there was nothing in the Act that stated that Congress would not have wanted the rest of the Act to stand had it known that states would have a genuine choice whether to participate in the new Medicaid expansion. For that reason, the court ruled that it must leave the rest of the Act intact.

Second Challenge

The case of <u>King v. Burwell</u> is expected to be argued before the United States Supreme Court in March 2015. This case is about how to construe a provision in the Affordable Care Act that every state must set up such an exchange. However, the statute later states that if a state elects not to set up an exchange the Department of Health and Human Services "shall . . . establish and operate such Exchange within the State."

The four italicized words imply that no tax credit is available at all for anyone enrolled in a plan obtained through an exchange set up by the federal government, because that's not an Exchange established by the State. Since 34 states declined to set up their own exchanges, most of the millions of people that everyone had assumed would be the law's beneficiaries are actually ineligible for the tax credit that was supposed to make their care affordable. It is certainly hoped that the United States Supreme Court will rule that the subsidy offered through an exchange established by Department of Health and Human Services can be granted.

CHAPTER 36

RECOGNITION OF SAME-SEX MARRIAGE FOR PURPOSES OF FEDERAL
LAW AND FLORIDA LAW

- Recognition of Same-Sex Marriage for Purposes of Federal
  Law and Regulations
- Recognition of Same-Sex Marriage for Purposes of Florida Law
- Supreme Court of United States to Review Circuit Split

Recognition of Same-Sex Marriage for Purposes of Federal Law and Regulations

The Federal Defense of Marriage Act (DOMA) was enacted by Congress in 1996 to define marriage as between one man and one woman for purposes of federal law and regulations. In particular, section 2 of DOMA, provides that one state cannot be required to give effect to the law of another state that recognizes any form of same-sex relationship or marriage. Section 3, defines the word "marriage" as between one man and one woman and "spouse" as someone of the opposite sex.

However, in 2013, the Supreme Court of the United States handed down the landmark case of U.S. v. Windsor, which held that section 3 of DOMA was unconstitutional under the Fifth Amendment of the United States Constitution. 133 S. Ct. 2675 (U.S. 2013). The Supreme Court did not address section 2 of DOMA because it was not challenged. In Windsor, Edith Windsor and Thea Spyer were lawfully married in Ontario, Canada in 2007 and then returned home to New York, which recognized the marriage as valid. Spyer died in 2009 and left her entire estate to Windsor. When Windsor claimed the marital deduction for surviving spouses under federal law, the exemption was denied under section 3 of DOMA. Windsor paid the taxes but challenged the constitutionality of the law.

In its opinion, the Supreme Court noted that traditionally marriage has been defined and regulated by the states and that the federal government deferred to state law. However, the Supreme Court further noted that the federal government had departed from this policy of deference to state law by enacting DOMA. The Supreme Court reasoned that the Congressional purpose of DOMA was to express moral disapproval of same-sex marriage by denying over 1000 federal benefits to legally married same-sex couples. Further, the Supreme Court stated that the primary effect of DOMA was to make same-sex marriages second class after traditional marriages. Therefore, the Supreme Court concluded that section 3 of DOMA violated Equal Protection and Due Process under the Fifth Amendment because the purpose and effect of the law was to injure a class of people that some states had sought to protect by legalizing same-sex marriage.

The Supreme Court issued an additional decision regarding same-sex marriage in Hollingsworth v. Perry, in which the constitutionality of California's Proposition 8 was challenged. 133 S. Ct. 2652 (U.S. 2013). In Hollingsworth, the controversy began when the California Supreme Court held that the exclusion of same sex-couples from marriage violated the Equal Protection Clause of the California Constitution. In response to the decision of the California Supreme Court, voters passed a referendum titled Proposition 8, which nominally excluded same-sex couples from marriage. However, California law continued to provide for "same-sex partnerships," which were treated in exactly the same manner and afforded all the same legal rights as heterosexual marriages. In a second California Supreme Court case, the Court held that the nominal exclusion of same-sex couples from marriage under Proposition 8 did not violate the Equal Protection because same-sex partnerships afforded same-sex couples substantially all of the same legal protections enjoyed by heterosexual married couples.

When the decision of the California Supreme Court to uphold Proposition 8 was challenged in a Federal District Court, it was found to violate the Equal Protection Clause of Fourteenth Amendment to the United States Constitution. The District Court reasoned, similar to Windsor, that there was no legitimate governmental purpose of Proposition 8 and held that it was unconstitutional.

The State of California refused to appeal the District Court's decision. Instead, the private group that organized Proposition 8 appealed the decision. When the appeal reached the Supreme Court, it determined that this group lacked standing to argue the case because it did not have a direct stake in the outcome. In other words, the private group had not suffered any direct injury; rather they were a group of citizens concerned about the law. Therefore, the Supreme Court dismissed the case without addressing its merits.

The decision of the Supreme Court in Windsor paved the way for same-sex couples to receive federal benefits for married couples. However, the ability of same-sex couples to receive federal benefits may depend on whether the couple lives in a state that recognizes same sex-marriage (recognition state) or a state that prohibits its recognition (non-recognition state). There is nothing standing in the way of same-sex couples receiving federal benefits when a same sex couple marries in a recognition state and lives in that state as their primary place of residence when they apply for federal benefits. In this type of case, federal agencies will recognize that the couple is married under that state's laws and thus married for purposes of receiving federal benefits.

The problem arises where a couple is lawfully married in a recognition state, but then moves to a non-recognition state. In this situation, Federal agencies follow either the "State of Celebration Rule" or the "State of Residence Rule." Under the State of Celebration Rule, the federal agency looks at the laws of the state in which the marriage was celebrated to determine whether a same-sex couple is validly married. However, under the State of Residence Rule, the federal agency looks at the laws of the state in which the same-sex couple resides to determine whether their marriage is valid.

The following paragraphs offer a brief summary of the policies that have been adopted by several Federal agencies and that have an impact on elder law and estate planning: The IRS issued Revenue Ruling 2013-17, which offers guidance on the application of Windsor to the Internal Revenue Code. In this ruling, the IRS adopted the State of Celebration Rule. In particular, the Service held that a same-sex marriage is valid if entered into in a state that recognizes same-sex marriage, even if the couple moves to a state that does not recognize same sex marriage. The IRS also clarified that gender specific terms (i.e., husband and wife) will be interpreted as gender neutral in order to include same-sex couples.

As a result of this Ruling, same-sex spouses who were married in a recognition state, even if they live in a non-recognition state, will be able to employ the spousal exemption from estate tax and other provisions of the Internal Revenue Code that apply to spouses in order to avoid Federal estate taxes.

Although the Social Security Administration (SSA) rules governing recognition of same-sex marriage for purposes of receiving SSA benefits are complex, the SSA has adopted the State of Residence Rule in regards to claims for the social security spousal benefit. See POMS GN 00210.003.

The SSA has adopted the State of Residence Rule regarding eligibility for federal Medicare benefits.

The Centers for Medicare & Medicaid Services (CMS) has clarified that pursuant to Windsor and Revenue Ruling 2013-17 same-sex couples who purchase insurance on the Federally-facilitated Marketplace are eligible for advance payments of premium tax credits and cost-sharing reductions. The State of Celebration Rule will be used to determine whether the marriage is valid.

The CMS has further clarified that although the federal government has adopted the IRS position (the State of Celebration Rule) for Medicaid purposes, non-recognition states are permitted to determine whether they will recognize marriages celebrated lawfully in recognition states in determining financial eligibility for Medicaid.

Pursuant to the United States Code, the VA follows a modified State of Residence Rule. The VA will recognize a same-sex marriage to be valid if (1) the veteran or spouse resided in a recognition state at the time of their marriage or (2) the veteran or spouse resides in a recognition state at the time the claim is filed.

The Department of Defense and the Military have adopted the State of Celebration Rule.

Recognition of Same-Sex Marriage for Purposes of Florida Law

The Florida Constitution and the Florida Statutes, similar to the federal DOMA, define marriage as between one woman and one man and prohibit recognition of same-sex marriages celebrated in other states.

Notwithstanding, in 2014, in the consolidated cases of <u>Brenner v. Scott</u> and <u>Grimsley v. Scott</u> ("<u>Brenner</u>"), the United States District Court for the North District of Florida held that the provisions of the Florida Constitution and the Florida Statutes banning same-sex marriage are unconstitutional under the Fourteenth Amendment of the United States Constitution.

In <u>Brenner</u>, the plaintiffs were several same-sex couples who had been denied marriage licenses by the Clerk of Court in their respective counties. The Court reasoned that Florida's ban on same-sex marriage violated Due Process and Equal Protection under the Fourteenth Amendment of the United States Constitution because the State of Florida did not have a sufficient reason to deny same-sex couples the fundamental right to marry. The Court granted a preliminary injunction, which ordered the officers of the State of Florida to cease enforcement of Florida's ban on same-sex marriage. The Court stayed the preliminary injunction pending appeals to the Eleventh Circuit Court of Appeals and the Supreme Court of the United States and 91 days thereafter.

Appeals to the Eleventh Circuit Court of Appeals and the Supreme Court of the United States were unsuccessful and the stay expired on January 6, 2015. Accordingly, same-sex marriage is now legal throughout the State of Florida, and Florida Clerks of Court have begun issuing marriage licenses to same-sex couples.

The impact of recognition of same-sex marriage in Florida is that, first, same-sex couples who are married in Florida (or who were validly married in another state but now reside in Florida) will now be eligible for Federal benefits without concern as to whether a particular federal agency may be following the State of Residence Rule in determining whether the couple is validly married for purposes of federal benefits.

In addition, same-sex couples can avail themselves of important state laws that impact married couples, such as the health care proxy provisions under the Florida Statutes, alimony and equitable division of assets upon dissolution of marriage, and elective share rights, family allowance, and exempt property provisions under the Florida Probate Code.

Supreme Court of United States to Review Circuit Split

In November of 2014, the Sixth Circuit Court of Appeals upheld bans on same-sex marriage in Ohio, Tennessee, Michigan, and Kentucky. This decision came in direct conflict with decisions of the Circuit Courts of Appeal for the Fourth, Seventh, Ninth, and Tenth Circuits.

In January of 2015, the Supreme Court granted certiorari regarding the decision of the Sixth Circuit Court of Appeals in order to resolve the conflict among the Circuit Courts.

The significance of decision of the Supreme Court to review the case is that the outcome will either determine that the States are free to enforce bans on same-sex marriage or that such bans are indeed in violation of the principles of Due Process and Equal Protection under the Fourteenth Amendment of the United States Constitution.

Accordingly, until the Supreme Court reaches its holding, the decision of the District Court for the Northern District of Florida in Brenner, finding that the Florida same-sex marriage ban is unconstitutional, is somewhat tentative because the Supreme Court could find on the contrary that the States are free to enact and enforce such bans, though such an outcome may be unlikely given the Supreme Court's holding in Windsor.

GLOSSARY

ADVANCE DIRECTIVES. These legal instruments permit an individual to express his or her treatment preferences in the event the person creating the document subsequently lacks the physical or mental capacity to make health care decisions. These documents include but are not limited to living wills, health care surrogate designations, pre-need guardian designations.

ANCILLARY ADMINISTRATION. Since the Florida courts have no jurisdiction over real property outside the boundaries of this state, the Florida personal representative (executor) does not have the authority to control the administration or management of real property in another state. Instead, the beneficiaries of that real property in another state must request that the court where the real property is located to open a second or ancillary probate proceeding. Likewise, there must be a second or ancillary administration of real property in Florida that is owned by a person who died a resident of another state.

ANATOMICAL GIFT. A person may make a gift of his or her body or body parts that will be effective at his or her death. The donation of a body or a body part must be to a hospital, a medical or dental school, a storage facility for medical or dental education, research or transplantation.

ANNUITANT. The person on which the annuity calculations are based. When the annuitant attains a certain age, the periodic payments begin.

ANNUITY. This is a contractual agreement whereby a person receives a lump sum in exchange for another's promise to pay a portion of the amount initially deposited together with interest over a term of years.

ASSIGNMENT. This is the procedure whereby a physician agrees to accept the Medicare-approved amount as full payment for his or her services.

BAKER ACT. This is a Florida statute intended to provide intense, short-term treatment for a person suffering with a mental, emotional, or behavioral disorder. This statute also authorizes continued treatment if it is necessary to assist a person in assuming responsibility for his or her treatment and recovery.

BALANCED BILL. A Medicare-approved physician not accepting assignment for payment of a Medicare claim may submit a balanced bill that does not exceed 115 percent of the Medicare-approved amount.

CLAIM. A person claiming that a deceased owes him or her a debt must file a claim with the clerk of the court in the county where the estate of the deceased person is being probated. The claim must be filed within the later of three months after notice to creditors was first published in the newspaper or within 30 days after the personal representative notifies a known creditor. If no notice to creditors is published and no notice is received from the personal representative, the claim must be filed with the clerk of the court within two years of the death of the debtor. If the claim is not timely filed, the enforcement of the debt may be barred.

CUSTODIAL CARE. This is level of care not requiring skilled nursing or rehabilitation. It includes assistance with bathing, toileting and other personal care needs that does not require the services of a nurse, therapist, or other skilled provider.

DECEASED SPOUSE'S UNUSED EXCLUSION (DSUE). The amount of the deceased spouse's unused applicable exclusion amount can be used by the surviving spouse against his or her estate tax if a portability exclusion is timely elected on the deceased spouse's estate tax return.

DEFERRED GIVING. A person may commit today to make a gift of property to a charity in the future. The person making the gift does this by signing an agreement that declares the property will pass to the charity at a future date. Until that time, the person who made the future gift to the charity or some other person may receive the income from this property.

DELEGABLE RIGHTS. If a person is determined by a circuit judge to be incapacitated in a guardianship proceeding, certain rights that the incapacitated person previously exercised may be removed and delegated to the guardian. These rights are to contract, sue and defend law suits, determine ones residency, consent to medical treatment, manage property, make gifts of property, or decide ones social environment. The judge then assigns the incapacitated persons delegable rights which are removed to a guardian.

DESIGNATED BENEFICIARY. This is the person named on the pension plan or Individual Retirement Account as the person(s) who will receive the balance of the pension plan or IRA that have not been distributed to the owner during lifetime. If there is no designated beneficiary, the balance will be paid to the deceased owner's estate.

DEVELOPMENTAL DISABILITY. This means a disorder or syndrome that is attributable to intellectual disability, cerebral palsy, autism, spina bifida, Prader-Willi Syndrome that manifests before age 18 and that constitutes a substantial handicap that can reasonably be expected to continue indefinitely.

DOCUMENTARY STAMP TAX. This money is paid to the Clerk of the Circuit Court in the county where a parcel of real property is situate before a deed transferring the ownership of that parcel of real property can be recorded in the Official Records of the Clerk of that court. This tax is also levied when a promissory note is given in exchange for a loan or when stock is issued.

DO-NOT-RESUSCITATE ORDER (DNRO). Resuscitation or life-prolonging techniques may be withheld or withdrawn from a patient by an emergency medical technician or paramedic if evidence of an order not to resuscitate by the terminal patients physician is presented to the emergency medical technician or paramedic. The DNRO form and patient identification device must be signed by the patient's physician. In addition, the patient, or, if the patient is incapable of providing informed consent, the patient's health care surrogate or proxy, or court appointed guardian or person acting pursuant to a durable power of attorney must sign the form and the patient identification device in order for them to be valid.

DURABLE POWER OF ATTORNEY. This instrument permits another person to serve as the agent for a person. The power of attorney is stated to be durable because it expressly states that the power of attorney is not affected by a subsequent incapacity of the principal.

ELECTIVE ESTATE. A surviving spouse is entitled to elect to receive 30 percent of the value of all the property of the deceased spouse wherever located, including joint accounts, pension benefits and in trust for accounts.

EXEMPT PROPERTY. The surviving spouse is entitled to $18,000 of household furniture and all automobiles used personally by the deceased spouse regardless of value. This is in addition to the elective estate and the family allowance.

EX PARTE ORDER. This order is issued by a Circuit Judge based on the affidavit of a physician or other health care physician stating that he or she has observed a person within the preceding 48 months who meets the criteria for involuntary examination. The order authorizes the Sheriff to take such a person to the nearest receiving facility for observation and treatment by a physician for up to 72 hours without a judicial hearing.

FAIR MARKET VALUE. The value of a home based on a comparison of that home with comparable homes in the same neighborhood that are either presently on the market or have sold in the last six months.

FEDERAL ESTATE TAX. This federal tax is imposed on transfers of property at death. An exception is made when the lifetime or death transfer is made to a qualified charity. The first $5.43 million of transfers at during lifetime and at death are excluded from this tax. This tax is 40% of the amount transferred in excess of the exclusion amount.

FEDERAL GENERATION TRANSFER TAX. There is another transfer tax that is imposed when the gift or devise is to a person in a generation that is more than one generation younger than the person making the transfer. The first $5.43 million of transfers are excluded from this tax. This tax is 40% of the amount transferred in excess of the exclusion amount.

FEDERAL GIFT TAX. This federal tax is imposed on transfers of property during lifetime. An exception is made when the lifetime or death transfer is made to a qualified charity. The first $5.43 million of transfers at during lifetime are excluded from this tax. This tax is 40% of the amount transferred in excess of the exclusion amount.

FREE LOOK PERIOD. All commercial annuities and insurance policies sold in Florida are required to have an unconditional refund period. The Florida statutes mandate a minimum of at least 10 days.

GATEKEEPER. A primary care physician assigned to an insured by a Health Maintenance Organization who must approve referrals to specialists within a health plan.

GIFT TAX ANNUAL EXCLUSION. This is the amount a person may give to another each year without filing a federal gift tax return form 709, or using any of his or her unified credit. Presently, a person may give up to $14,000 per person per year without filing a gift tax return or using his or her unified credit against gift or estate tax.

GRANDPARENT VISITATION. This refers to Court ordered visits by grandparents when a grandchild is experiencing significant mental or emotional harm due to the parental decision to prohibit grandparent visitation.

GUARDIANSHIP. This occurs when a circuit judge determines that a person lacks the capacity to manage his or her property or to meet at least some of the essential health and safety requirements. A person cannot manage his or her property if he or she is unable to take the necessary actions to obtain, administer and dispose of his or her real and personal property. A person cannot meet the essential requirements for health or safety if he or she cannot take the necessary actions to provide the health care, food, shelter, clothing, personal hygiene, or other care without possibly causing serious and immediate physical injury or illness to occur.

HEALTH CARE SURROGATE. A written document that can be signed in advance of an incapacity naming another person as a surrogate to make health care decisions. A health care surrogate has the authority to make all health care decisions for the person during a time of mental incapacity. A person may designate a separate surrogate to consent to mental health treatment in the event he or she is determined by a court to be incompetent to consent to mental health treatment and a guardian advocate is appointed.

HMO. Health Maintenance Organization

HOME EQUITY CONVERSION MORTGAGE. This is a reverse mortgage that is insured by the Federal Housing Administration. A reverse mortgage is a home loan that provides cash advances to a homeowner, but does not required any certain repayment until the home is sold or the homeowner dies or relocates.

HOME HEALTH CARE. Medicare Part A will pay for a limited amount of assistance if an insured is generally confined to the home (homebound) and the condition is such that the patient requires assistance to leave home (cane, walker, or assistance of another person, etc.) or that leaving the home without assistance is not advisable, or that leaving home requires a considerable effort, and the patient must require skilled care: either speech or physical therapy services or intermittent skilled nursing care.

HOMESTEAD TAX EXEMPTION. A tax credit for Florida residents on their principal residence.

HOSPICE. In order for a person to be entitled to Medicare Hospice coverage he or she must be certified as terminally ill. This means a physician must determine to a reasonable medical certainty that the person's life expectancy is six months or less if the illness follows its expected course. The primary advantage of hospice Medicare is that a terminal patient's broad needs can be met with a hidden array of services for a longer period of time. Hospice care provides the terminally ill patient with a holistic approach that concentrates on the patients pain management, offers specialized care, and attempts to meet the spiritual and emotional needs of the patient and his or her family.

INCOME CAP. This is the maximum amount of monthly income that the institutionalized spouse can receive and still be eligible for nursing home assistance. The monthly gross income available to the institutionalized spouse cannot exceed the state monthly income cap. However, a nursing home patient with a gross monthly income in excess of the income cap can still qualify for the institutional care program by establishing an irrevocable qualified income trust. This trust is often referred to as a Miller Trust, after the name of the Colorado case that originally approved this concept.

INTANGIBLE TAX. The amount paid to the Clerk of the Circuit Court when the mortgage is recorded in the Official Records.

INTESTATE. This is a probate proceeding for a person who dies a resident of Florida without leaving a valid will.

IRREVOCABLE TRUST. This cannot be amended or altered. The assets conveyed to an irrevocable trust cannot be withdrawn or returned to the grantor or settlor. An irrevocable trust is normally created for estate tax purposes.

LATE RETIREMENT. A Social Security insured worker who delays retirement until after he or she is eligible for full retirement benefits. The worker may receive increased benefits in two ways. First, the extra income earned after full retirement age usually increases average earnings because this later years earnings may replace a previous lower year of earnings. Secondly, a special credit is given to a worker who delays retirement.

LIVING WILL. A witnessed written document in which a person states whether a life-prolonging procedure would be withheld or withdrawn if his or her medical condition is determined to be terminal or a permanent vegetative state.

LIFE-PROLONGING PROCEDURE. Any medical procedure, treatment, or intervention which uses mechanical or other artificial means to sustain, restore, or replace a spontaneous vital function; and when applied to a patient in a terminal condition, serves only to prolong the dying process.

LIMITING CHARGE. A physician not accepting assignment for payment of a Medicare claim may submit a balance bill which does not exceed 115 percent of the Medicare approved amount.

LONG-TERM CARE INSURANCE. This can reimburse a person for subsequent expenses related to a stay in a nursing home, assisted living facility or for home health care.

MANAGED CARE PLAN. This involves a group of doctors, hospitals, and other health care providers who have agreed to provide care to Medicare beneficiaries in exchange for a fixed amount of money from Medicare. There are normally no deductibles or co-pays charged to the patient.

MARITAL DEDUCTION TRUST. This assures the surviving spouse the net income from the trust assets at least annually and as much of the assets of the trust necessary for the surviving spouse's health, education, maintenance and support. For the deceased's estate to be entitled to the marital deduction, the trust must also grant the surviving spouse a general power of appointment to state who will receive the remaining trust principal upon his or her death. In a marital deduction trust, the assets of the trust will not be subject to federal estate taxes when the first spouse dies, but will be taxed at the death of the second spouse.

MEDICARE. Congress approved Medicare in 1965 to provide health insurance for a person age 65 or older or permanently disabled and eligible for social security. Congress later amended these laws to extend coverage to disabled workers. The care and supplies must be medically reasonable and necessary for treatment or diagnosis. The care and supplies must be prescribed by a doctor. The services and the supplies must be obtained through a Medicare-certified provider.

MEDICARE PART A. This covers acute hospital care, a limited number of skilled nursing days, rehabilitation therapy, home health care and hospice care.

MEDICARE PART B. This covers payment of the physicians' charges. In addition, durable medical equipment, outpatient physical therapy, X-ray and diagnostic tests are also covered. Physicians agree to accept the Medicare approved amount as full payment. Medicare will pay 80% and the patient is responsible to pay the 20% co-payment.

MEDIGAP. The supplemental policy needed to cover the costs not provided by Medicare. The policies as sold by private companies.

MEDICARE & YOU. Medicare handbook explaining information about the variety of managed care plans available to them in geographic area. This handbook can be presently found on the Internet web site www.medicare.gov.

MEDICAID NURSING HOME ASSISTANCE. A nursing home patient may be eligible for assistance in paying a portion of his or her custodial nursing home cost through the State of Florida's institutional care program which is partially funded by Medicaid.

MONTHLY MINIMUM MAINTENANCE NEEDS INCOME ALLOWANCE. This is amount sometimes referred to as a MMMNIA. This is the amount of the institutionalized spouse's income that may be retained necessary to allow the community spouse a minimum income of per month. There may be an additional amount of income diverted from the institutionalized spouse if the community spouse can demonstrate excess shelter expenses.

MORTGAGE. A document that places a lien on real property. The lender holds the lien as security for their borrowed money.

PATIENT PAY AMOUNT. This is the amount paid to the nursing home by the patient. It is determined after first allowing the patient a monthly needs allowance of $105 per month and after first permitting the patient's spouse to receive the monthly minimum maintenance needs income allowance referred to above. The state of Florida then pays both nursing home the balance of the bill for the patient's care.

PATIENT PROTECTION AND AFFORDABLE CARE ACT. This new law permits new employees and /or family members of existing employees to be added to existing plans without losing the plan's grandfathered status. It provides for the inclusion of coverage for young adults and pre-existing conditions. Group Health Insurance Plans must provide unlimited coverage. The law provides for mandatory coverage without rescission. Beginning in 2014 a qualified health insurance plan will be offered through the American Health Benefit Exchange . Also, there will be a penalty assessed in 2014 that will be called a shared responsibility payment if a person does not purchase health insurance. However, abortion coverage is prohibited from being required as part of the essential health benefits package. The PPACA was determined to be constitutional by the United States Supreme Court in the summer of 2012.

PATIENT SELF-DETERMINATION ACT. This law requires hospitals, nursing homes, home health care agencies and hospice programs to develop policies and educational programs on advance directives for patients, staff and community.

PERSISTENT VEGETATIVE STATE. This is characterized by a permanent and irreversible condition of unconsciousness in which there is the absence of voluntary action or cognitive behavior and an inability to communicate or interact with the environment.

PERSONAL REPRESENTATIVE: The person appointed by the court to administer the estate. This person manages the deceased's assets and later distributes the probate assets to the beneficiaries.

PERSONAL SERVICE CONTRACT. A period of Medicaid ineligibility will usually not result if the person in need of assistance initially contracts with a family member or a friend prior to these personal services being rendered. In such event, real or personal property estimated to equal the value of the services to be rendered to the infirmed person can be transferred in exchange for an agreement to provide the personal services over the infirmed person's lifetime.

PET TRUST. A trust for the care of a deceased person's animals.

PORTABILITY. This is the term used for the surviving spouse using the last deceased spouse's unused exemption equivalent to offset the surviving spouse's estate tax.

POSTNUPTIAL AGREEMENT. This can be signed by spouses after the marriage to waive some or all marital rights. The purpose of this agreement is to promote each individuals mutual welfare and happiness in the marriage and to avoid disharmony, misunderstanding and uncertainty during the marriage or after the marriage ends because of divorce, death or other causes. The agreement provides that each spouse solely retains his or her assets and income.

PREMATURE DISTRIBUTION. This will occur when a participant in a retirement plan or an owner of an IRA receives a distribution of money from the retirement plan or IRA before the age of 59 1/2. Unless there is an exception, the IRS penalizes a premature distribution with an additional 10 percent excise tax.

PRENUPTIAL AGREEMENT. Spouses considering a second marriage should also consider signing a prenuptial agreement. The purpose of this agreement is to promote each individuals mutual welfare and happiness in the marriage and to avoid disharmony, misunderstanding and uncertainty during the marriage or after the marriage ends because of divorce, death or other causes. The agreement provides that each spouse solely retains his or her assets and income.

PROBATE. The purpose of probate is to collect a deceased persons assets, pay his or her claims, taxes and administrative expenses from these assets, and distribute the remainder of the assets administrative expenses to the beneficiaries entitled to receive them. A personal representative (known as an executor) is appointed by the court to pay the deceased's claims and taxes and to distribute the remainder of the estate assets according to the terms of the deceased persons will.

QUALIFIED INCOME TRUST. This trust is often referred to as a Miller Trust originally the name of the Colorado case which initially approved this concept. The irrevocable trust must consist of only the patient's income and the earnings on the income. In essence, the patient or a representative deposits into this irrevocable trust the excess portion of his or her income which is at least the amount that will cause the patient to be considered to have available income of less than the income cap.

QUALIFIED TERMINAL INTEREST TRUST (or Q-TIP TRUST). This trust also qualifies for the estate tax marital deduction if the deceased's personal representative makes the Q-tip election on the deceased's estate tax return. The surviving spouse only receives the net income earned from the assets placed in this trust at least annually. At the death of the surviving spouse, the assets in the trust are paid to a beneficiary previously named by the first spouse before his or her death.

REQUIRED DISTRIBUTION. A participant of a pension plan or an IRA must begin receiving distributions by the time he or she reaches the Required Beginning Date. The Required Beginning Date normally cannot exceed the first day in April of the year following the calendar year in which the participant is 70 1/2.

REVOCABLE TRUST. This is an agreement established during lifetime. The person establishing the agreement has the right during lifetime to convey assets to the trustee of this agreement or to request a return of the assets. This agreement can be cancelled or changed during the lifetime of the person creating the agreement. The trust becomes irrevocable upon the death of the person establishing the agreement. The assets pass at death to named beneficiaries without probate proceedings.

ROTH IRA. The contributions accumulate tax free and qualified distributions from that IRA will be income tax free. The contributions to the Roth IRA, however, are not tax deductible.

SETTLOR. A settlor or grantor is a person creating the trust.

SKILLED NURSING FACILITY CARE. These facilities provide skilled nursing services that are received by a patient on a daily basis which means therapy services at least five days per week and nursing care seven days per week.

SOCIAL SECURITY. A national program which pay benefits received by the retired and disabled workers, their spouses, their dependents, widows, widowers or children of deceased workers.

SOCIAL SECURITY LIMITS ON EARNINGS. There is no limit on earnings for a person receiving social security who is over age 65. Between 62 and 66, there is a reduction in Social Security benefits. For every $2 earned over the limit, $1 is withheld from Social Security benefits.

SOCIAL SECURITY DISABILITY INSURANCE (SSDI). A worker must be under 65; disabled and have obtained a status of disability insured or specially insured by the Social Security Administration.

SPRINGING DURABLE POWER OF ATTORNEY. Previously, a person could condition the effective date of a durable power of attorney upon his or her actually becoming incapacitated. This amendment to the Florida statute stated that the durable power of attorney can be conditioned upon the person creating this durable power of attorney lacking the capacity to manage property as defined in the Florida guardianship statute. Effective October 1, 2011, a springing durable power of attorney cannot be created. Existing springing durable power of attorneys created prior to that date are still valid.

TERMINAL CONDITION. This means a person is suffering from:

A. A condition caused by injury, disease, or illness from which there is no reasonable probability of recovery and which, without treatment, can be expected to cause death, or

B. A persistent vegetative state characterized by a permanent and irreversible condition of unconsciousness in which there is the absence of voluntary action or cognitive behavior or an inability to communicate or interact with the environment, or

C. An end-state stage condition

TESTAMENTARY TRUST. A trust established in a Last Will and Testament, which becomes effective upon the death of the person executing the will. A testamentary trust is important for the parent of minor children. Florida law permits a child to receive his or her deceased parents' assets at age 18, unrestricted from guardianship supervision. A testamentary trust can provide for the retaining of these assets by a trustee until the child has attained a more mature age.

TESTATOR OR TESTATRIX. The person creating the will. A man is referred to as the testator. A woman is referred to as the testatrix.

TITLE INSURANCE. To reimburse the buyer of the real property or the owner of a mortgage against a loss in the event the title to the real property is subsequently to be determined to be defective or invalid.

TRUST. A trust which is established during the lifetime of the person creating the trust is a revocable trust permits the grantor or settlor to revoke the trust, alter the terms of the trust, or withdraw some or all of the assets from the trust. A revocable trust becomes irrevocable at the death of the grantor or settlor. A testamentary trust is a trust created at death in a Last Will and Testament.

UNEARNED INCOME MEDICARE CONTRIBUTION TRUST. Starting in 2013, the new Health Care legislation imposes an additional Unearned Income Medicare Contributions Tax (UIMCT) equal to 3.8% of the lesser of the net investment income or the excess of the modified adjusted gross income over the applicable threshold dividends, annuities, royalties, rents, net gain from property held for investment over the applicable threshold amount. The threshold amount will be $200,000 for individuals and $250,000 in a year for a married couple.

VIATICAL AGREEMENTS. A person or a privately owned company agrees to purchase a life insurance policy or a portion of the life insurance policy's face value from a person who has a catastrophic or life-threatening illness or condition. The owner of the policy can expect to receive a percentage of the policy's face value, depending on:(a) his or her projected life expectancy; (b) the projected cost of the remaining premiums due before death; (c) the time value of money.

WILL. A legal document signed by the person intending to give his or her assets at death to others. Two witnesses must attest that person's signature by signing in the document in his presence and in the presence of each other.

Index

A

Adult Family-Care Home 93, 94
  Define 93
  License 93
Advance Directives 59, 60, 73, 193
  Do-not-resuscitate order 71, 195
  Health Care 59
  Living Wills 59, 198
  Patient Self-Determination Act 59, 201
Annuitant 41, 42, 43, 44, 45, 46, 47, 49, 109, 110, 193
  Designated Beneficiary Form 42
Annuities 5,6, 41, 43, 44, 45, 46, 48, 49, 103, 108, 109, 155, 159
  Estate Taxation of Annuities 41
  Inappropriate Sale Practices 47
Annuitization Date 41, 42
  Death of Owner 42
  Deferred Annuities 44, 46, 48
  Distribution of 42
  Fixed Deferred Annuity 44
  Free Look Period 45, 196
  Immediate Annuities 43
  Income Taxation of 45
  Life Income Annuity 43
  Life with Period Certain 43
  Maturity Date 41
  Owner 41, 42, 44, 45, 46, 49
  Penalty for Early Withdrawal 45
  Variable Deferred Annuity 44
Annuity 41-49, 108, 109,110, 113, 157, 158,159, 160, 193
Assisted Living Facility 79, 82, 93, 94, 115, 116, 121, 125, 127
Assisted Living Facility Medicaid Waiver Program 114
Attorney Fees 130, 162
  Compensation 163
  Extraordinary 163
  Ordinary Services 163

B

Baker Act 81, 83, 193
  Adult Day Care Center 82, 83
  Assisted Living Facility 82
  Circuit Judge 81, 82
  Clinical Psychologist 81, 82
  Consent to Treatment 81, 82, 83
  Crisis Service 82
  Examination 81, 82
  Ex-Parte Order 81
  Guardian Advocate 81, 82, 83
  Human Rights 81
  Initial Assessment 82
  Involuntary Commitment 82
  Involuntary Placement 81, 82
  Involuntary Psychiatric Examination 81
  Law Enforcement Officer 81, 82
  Licensed Clinical Social Worker 81
  Mental Health Facility 81, 82
  Mental Health Treatment 81, 83
  Mental Illness 81, 83
  Nursing Home 82
  Petition for Involuntary Placement 82
  Physician 81, 82
  Psychiatric Nurse 81
  Receiving or Treatment Facility 82
  Training Course 83
  Writ of Habeas Corpus 82

C

Charitable Remainder Annuity Trust (CRAT) 157, 158
Charitable Remainder Trust 155, 157, 158
Charitable Remainder Unitrust (CRUT) 157, 158
Codicil 135, 136, 170

D

Disabled Adult 93, 99, 100, 101
Documentary Stamp Tax 54, 195
Do-Not-Resuscitate Order (DNRO) 71, 195
  CPR 71
  Department of Health 71, 93
  Doctor's Order 71
  Emergency Medical Service 71
Durable Power of Attorney 60, 75, 76, 77, 79, 88, 89, 90, 119, 195
  Affidavit 76, 78
  Agent 75, 76, 77, 78
  Guardian 75, 78
  Pets 79
  Revoked 75
  Springing Durable Power of Attorney 76, 203
  Suspended 75
  Terminated 75, 77

E

Elder Abuse 99

Adult Protective Services Act 99
Central Abuse Registry 99, 100
Civil or Criminal Liability 99
Department of Children and Families 99, 100, 101
Disabled Person 99, 100, 101
Exploitation 99, 100, 101, 102
Fine 100, 101
Protective Service Investigator 100
Toll Free Telephone Number 99
Elder Mediation 127, 128
Elective Estate 146, 147, 148, 195

F

Federal Estate and Gift Tax Law 149
Alternate Valuation Date 151
Annual Exclusion 149, 154
Gross Estate 149, 150, 151
Step-Up-In-Basis 151
Taxable Estate 151, 153
Free Look Period 45, 196
Funeral Arrangements 167, 168
Cremation 167, 168
Organ Donation 167, 170
Pre-Need Arrangements 167
Pre-Need Funeral Provider 167
Prepaid Burial 167
Right-to-rescind 167
Waiting Period 169

G

Gift Annuity 159, 160
Grandparent Visitation 131, 196
Health and Welfare of the Child 131
Parental Rights 131
Troxel v. Granville 131
Guardian 60, 63, 64, 71, 73, 75, 78, 82, 86, 90, 97, 98, 101, 114
Guardianships 85, 197
Bond 86
Circuit Judge 85, 86
Examining Committee 85
Incapacitated 85, 86
Licensed Social Worker 85
Petition to Determine the Incapacity 86
Psychologist 85
Registered Nurse 85

H

Health Care Proxy 64, 70, 73, 190
Health Care Surrogate 60, 63, 64, 69, 70, 71, 73, 79, 82, 83, 86, 89, 90, 146, 171, 197

Holographic Will 135
Hospice 16, 20, 21, 24, 25, 59, 67, 71, 116, 177, 197

I

Individual Retirement Account (IRA) 29-40
Contribution Limit 29, 38
Designated Beneficiary 31, 32, 33, 34, 36, 40, 47, 108, 158, 194
Educational Expenses 30
Estate Taxation 29, 40
First Home 38
Medical Expenses 30
Minimum Distribution 31, 32, 36, 37
Required Distributions 29, 31, 39, 202
Roth IRA 29, 35, 37, 38, 39, 40, 203
Traditional 31, 34, 35, 37, 38, 39, 40
Intangible Tax 55, 198

L

Life-Prolonging Procedure 61, 62, 198
Living Wills 59, 61, 63, 64, 198
Absence of a Living Will 61, 63
Bush v. Schiavo 64
Elective Procedures 61, 62
End-Stage Condition 61, 62, 64
Exercising a Living Will 61, 62
In re Guardianship of Schiavo 64
Irreversible Condition 61
Life-Prolonging Procedure 61, 62, 198
McIver v. Krischer 65
Mercy Killing 61, 65
Persistent Vegetative State 61, 64, 73, 201

M

Medicaid 103, 104, 105, 107, 109-118
60-Month Look-Back Period 112
Burial Contract 104
Eligibility 104, 105, 108, 109, 115, 116
Exemptions to the Transfer Rules 112
Irrevocable Annuities 108
Irrevocable Qualified Income Trust 104
Life Expectancy Tables 105, 108, 109
Look-Back Period 107, 111, 126
Personal Service Contract 110, 111, 201
Supplemental Needs Trust 112, 113, 114
Medicaid Estate Recovery Act 116
Medicare 15-28, 199
Home Health Care 15, 16, 18, 19, 197
Part A 15, 16, 17, 18, 21, 199
Part B 15, 16, 17, 18, 21, 22, 23, 199
Part D 15, 24, 25, 26, 27, 28

Reasonable Charge 22
Skilled Nursing Facility Care 16, 18, 203

N

Net Income Charitable Remainder Unitrust (NICRUT) 158
Net Income With Make-up Charitable Remainder Unitrust (NIMCRUT) 158
Nuncupative Will 135
Nursing Home 95, 96, 97, 98
    Appeals 96
    Basis for Discharge 95
    Discharges 95, 96
    Emergency Discharge 97
    Patient Rights 95
    Resident's Rights 95, 97
    Transfer 95, 96, 97, 98

O

Office of the Local Long-Term Care Ombudsman 98

P

Pension Plan 29, 30, 31, 38, 39, 40
  Distribution 29-40
  Distributions Upon Participant's Death Before Required Beginning Date 29, 32
  Minimum Distributions 31, 32, 36, 37
  Premature Distributions 29, 30, 201
  Required Distributions 29, 31, 39, 202
  Rollover by Surviving Spouse 29, 33
  Roth IRA 29, 35, 37, 38, 39, 40, 203
  Trust as Beneficiary 29, 36
Personal Representative 80, 98, 116, 136, 150, 151, 152, 161, 162, 163, 201
Pets 79
  Prepay Medical Care 80
  Provide for Exercise, Grooming, Veterinary Care and Special Dietary Needs 80
Pooled Income Fund 155, 160
Postnuptial Agreement 146, 201
Power of Attorney 75, 76, 77, 78
Pre-Need Guardian 86
Prenuptial Agreement 145, 146, 201
Probate 161, 162, 163, 164, 165, 202
  Alternatives to Formal Probate 163
  Automobile 164
  Department of Motor Vehicles 164, 165
  Disposition Without Need of Administration 164
Prostate Screening 21

Q

Qualified Terminal Interest Trust (Q-TIP trust) 202

R

Resident's Bill of Rights 94

S

Self-Proved Will 136
Selling a Residence 51
  Capital Gain 51, 52
  Florida Documentary Stamp 51, 54
  Principal Residence 51, 53
  Title Insurance 55, 204
Social Security 3-14, 203
  Delayed Retirement Credit 8
  Determining Disability 13
  Disability Benefits and Eligibility 12
  Disabled Widow's/Widower's Benefits 13
  Divorced Spouse's Benefits 10
  Early Retirement 6, 7, 8
  Family Benefits 11, 14
  Full Retirement 4, 6, 7, 8, 10
  Late Retirement 8, 198
  Limits on Earnings 4
  Married Spouse's Benefits 10
  Parent's Benefits 12
  Regular Retirement 5, 6, 7, 8, 9
  Social Security Taxes 4
  Surviving Spouse's Benefits 11
  Taxation of 9
Standard Charitable Remainder Unitrust 158
Step-Up-in-Basis 151

T

Title Insurance 51, 55, 204
Trusts 139, 142
  Beneficiaries 139, 141, 143, 157
  Creditors 141, 142
  Grantor 139, 140, 141, 142, 143
  Homestead Tax Exemption 140, 197
  Irrevocable 139, 140, 141, 142
  Living Trust 139, 140, 142
  Pour-Over Will 139
  Revocable 139, 140, 143, 202
  Settlor 139, 140, 141, 142, 203
  Successor Trustee 139, 140, 141
  Summary Probate Administration 141
  Trustee 139, 140, 141, 142, 143

V

Veterans 173, 174, 176, 177, 179
  Benefits 173, 174, 176, 177
  Cemeteries 179
  Gravesite 179
  Headstone 179
  Internment in a National Cemetery 179
Viatical Agreements 129, 130, 204
Department of Insurance 129
  Policyholder 129, 130
Viatical Settlement Provider 129, 130

W

Wills 135
  Codicil 135, 136, 170
  Executor 136
  Handwritten 135
  Holographic 135
  Importance of Having Signed and Witnessed 135
  Intestate 135, 198
  Nuncupative 135
  Probate 135, 136, 137

ORDER FORM

Fax orders to: (727) 499-6937

Telephone orders to: Toll free: 1-888-298-8115

Postal orders: PO Box 733
                       New Port Richey, FL 34656

Name: _____

Company: _____

Address: _____

City: _____ State: _____ Zip: _____

Please send me _____ copies of The Florida Senior Legal Guide 9th Edition:
@ 39.95 per book.

Please send me _____ copies of The Florida Senior Legal Guide 9th Edition
DVD @ $19.95 per DVD.

_____ books @ $39.95 each = $ _____
_____ DVD's @ $19.95 each = $ _____
7% Sales tax (Florida residents only) $ _____
Shipping & Handling: $7.50 each book/$5.00 $ _____
Each DVD
                              TOTAL $ _____

Payment Method:

Check (make check payable to Senior Law Series, Inc.)
Credit Card: Visa   MasterCard

Name on card: _____
Card Number: _____
CVV2/CID (3 or 4 digits on back of card)_____
Expiration Date: _____

or you may purchase on line at
www.seniorlawseries.com